MW01109095

FOOD ISN'T WHAT IT USED TO BE

A BIBLICAL APPROACH TO HEALTH

To your health!

Christine Andrew

By:

Christine Andrew, CNC

Food Isn't What It Used To Be
Copyright © 2016 by Christine Andrew, CNC

All rights reserved. No part of this publication may be reproduced, distributed, or transmitted in any form or by any means, including photocopying, recording, or other electronic or mechanical methods, without the prior written permission of the publisher or author, except in the case of brief quotations embodied in critical reviews and certain other noncommercial uses permitted by copyright law.

Although every precaution has been taken to verify the accuracy of the information contained herein, the author and publisher assume no responsibility for any errors or omissions. No liability is assumed for damages that may result from the use of information contained within.

All scriptural references are with New King James version unless otherwise noted.

Library of Congress Control Number: 2012924322
ISBN-13:   Paperback: 978-1-68256-732-6
           PDF: 978-1-68256-733-3
           ePub: 978-1-68256-734-0
           Kindle: 978-1-68256-735-7
           Hardcover   978-1-68256-736-4

Printed in the United States of America

LitFire LLC
1-800-511-9787
www.litfirepublishing.com
order@litfirepublishing.com

CONTENTS

Recipes

"Food Isn't What It Used To Be" is a great read! Christine does a wonderful job of harmonizing Biblical truths, leading-edge medical science and common sense lifestyle modifications. Following these principles can add years to your life and life to your years!

KC Craichy-Author: The Super Health Diet
- The Last Diet You Will Ever Need!

Christine's depth of knowledge and passion for helping people is evident in her writing. Her writing conveys her desire to help others find the best sources of nutrition available. The reader will be challenged by this thought provoking work, and will be inspired to make healthy life changes based on her research as it align with God's word.

Kimberly A. Floyd, MA, Educator

DISCLAIMER

The information and recommendations outlined in this book are not intended as a substitute for personalized medical advice. The presentation proposes certain theoretical methods of nutrition not necessarily mainstream. It is left to the discretion and it is the sole responsibility of the user of the information indicated in the presentation to determine if procedures and recommendations described are appropriate for a patient. The presenter of this information cannot be held responsible for the information or any inadvertent errors or omissions of the information.

The information in this presentation should not be construed as a claim or representation that any procedure or product mentioned constitutes a specific cure, palliative or ameliorative. Procedures described should be considered as adjunctive to other accepted conventional procedures deemed necessary by the attending licensed doctor.

It is the concern of the Department of Health and Human Services that no homeopathic and nutritional supplements be used to replace established, conventional medical approaches, especially in cases of emergencies, serious or life-threatening diseases, or conditions.

I share in this concern especially in serious cases. Replacing conventional treatment with alternative methods could deprive the patient of necessary treatment and cause harm as well as posing a major legal liability for the health professional involved. No supplement formula should be used as a replacement for conventional medical treatment.

-Christine Andrew
Certified Nutrition Consultant

Acknowledgements

I wish to thank my mentor and friend, William Kneebone, DC who gave me the original inspiration to write this book and who instilled in me tremendous knowledge in the field of nutrition and health. He will be forever missed. It is to him I wish to dedicate this book.

I wish to also thank my sister, Kathrine Page, for all her knowledge and valuable theological contributions to this book. Abundant gratitude and thanks to Nancy Miller and Kimberly Floyd who worked diligently editing and revising the first printing of this book. Their advice added immense benefit to this manuscript. Thank you David Stewart, PhD for your encouragement in writing this book.

I want to thank my maternal grandparents and my mother for instilling in my roots the value of home grown foods, home cooking, sustainable farming practices, and healthy eating habits. Although there was a period of time that I strayed from the lessons taught, I would not be where I am today in my health if it were not for the foundational lessons passed down from my ancestors.

I wish to thanks the many friends for their prayers and encouragement in the writing of this book. Cory, Karen, Lee and Mary, Crystal, Kim, my pastor Jon, and many others, thank you for your confidence in me and for your encouragement.

Current research and added recipes inspired me to write a second edition of this book.

INTRODUCTION

Food Isn't What it Used to Be

Death is inevitable; it always has been. Since the Garden of Eden, we've lived in a fallen world. Adam lived in a perfect world. There was no sickness or death. Because of Adam's fall, we were to forever experience disease, pain, and death this side of heaven. While our appointed time to die is only known by God, it is our responsibility, while living, to take care of the body He has entrusted to us. We take great care, time and effort in caring for our cars, houses, yards, and churches, but how many give thought to how we truly care for our physical bodies? When our car breaks down, we buy a new one; when our plants die, we buy new ones, but when our health declines, we seek help from an industry that is guided by a monopoly that cares more about profits than the food we eat. Even though we have this appointed time, it is interesting to note that in ancient civilizations people lived well into the age of one hundred years or more. In comparison, it has been said that this generation today will not outlive their parents and this is clearly evidenced by the obituaries with younger and younger people dying and the staggering statistics of deaths worldwide reported by the CDC every year.

How is it that "medical care" was not advanced as today, food variety was scarce compared to today, yet people lived to advanced years? Michael Pollan in his newest book, *Food Rules*, reports that we are generally living longer than people used to, but most of our added years is owed to gains in infant mortality and child health, not diet.[34] We now have the most advanced health care in the nation with thousands of food choices, yet we are an unhealthy "sick" nation continuing to struggle with disease and death. Old diseases once thought conquered have reemerged. Antibiotic resistance has soared. New plagues never thought possible are emerging.

According to Dr. Bernard Jensen, "….when we read the FDA's familiar "Composition of Foods" chart to find out how much iron is in our sesame seeds or how much calcium is in our greens, these figures are completely irrelevant to today's food. They are derived from the "Firman Bear" report of 1963. The average nutritional values found in 1963 were already well below the lowest values in the previous study, from 1948." Imagine how much lower they've gone since that time! He continues, "At this point our foods may be virtually "empty."[20] In order to get the amount of iron obtained from one cup of spinach in 1945 takes 65 cups today. In order to obtain the 50 mg. of vitamin C found in an orange in 1950 requires 10 oranges today.[21] Something has dramatically changed in the last 4,000 years and even as recently as the last 50-60 years.

I was raised in a family where the food eaten was fresh and made from scratch. We ate meals together as a family. Fresh homemade lunches were taken to school daily. It was a rare occasion that we ate TV dinners, sweets, or soda. My mother, who learned from her mother, was the best cook ever. But growing up with peer pressure, I frequently felt deprived of the "good" food. After leaving home for college I found myself beginning to eat whatever tasted good, but still at the back of my mind I knew what I should eat. As the years progressed I feasted on fast food and packaged processed foods mainly for breakfasts and lunches. My favorite soda was Dr. Pepper or Root Beer. Dinners, however, were still home cooked with fresh vegetables and salads.

By the time I was 26 years old, I began to notice my first of several health challenges. Fatigue and shakiness overcame me if meals were missed, for which I was frequently guilty. The pain every month in my lower abdomen sent me doubled over motionless. After seeing four doctors who couldn't tell me what was happening and although never tested, my hormones had become quite out of balance, and I eventually was diagnosed with Endometriosis. The standard treatment at that time was a powerful and costly hormone drug. I continued for eleven years on that hormone treatment. The pain was gone but the impact of my health challenges roared its full head at 40 years old. At this point not only did the endometrial pain come back with a vengeance, digestive issues were constant. I was then diagnosed with IBS and no suggestions from doctors for how to help except to get off dairy.

It was about that time I decided to travel down my own health journey toward healing. I changed my diet, some, and began to take a few supplements. A year later it was imperative that I have surgery for the endometriosis. However, my health had not been restored through this treatment. Two years later a brain tumor was discovered and subsequently removed. Digestive issues continued to worsen. Weight gained on me without notice. Doctors could not seem to help. After visiting a holistic healthcare practitioner, who later became my mentor for my nutrition internship program, I learned that I had leaky gut, gluten intolerance, and several other food sensitivities. We began a healing journey that took two years of hard work, perseverance through dietary changes and depression, prayer, and dedication to bring my health back into balance, yet has now stood the test of time. I will forever be grateful for having met my mentor who encouraged me in my field of nutrition and in the writing of this book.

Through my own health challenges I decided to dig deep into scripture to find out what the Bible had to say about health, disease, emotions, and remedies. If natural remedies worked since ancient times, surely it would be viable for today's standards. According to the FDA-Natural is defined as anything that ultimately comes from nature. God, the creator of nature, has defined certain things for us to eat and drink. The Bible always has been our source of information for everything we need. This includes fundamental principles for how to approach health. It was my quest to find out what exactly was eaten and consumed during the ancient times and to show how food choices, consumption, and health has truly changed throughout history and learn what we need to do to fulfill our calling.

I'd like to thank John MacArthur for his encouraging quote:
An uncompromising life is characterized by an unashamed boldness

that calls us to an uncommon standard. Allow God to do with your life as He pleases, that He might broaden your influence and glorify Himself.

It is my prayer and hope that through the boldness of this writing, you would broaden your knowledge about the importance of eating the right foods for health and that God would be honored and glorified.

1

. . . . . .

Created in God's Image

Just about anywhere you look today there are reports, books, magazines, and news articles about health. Yet you look at doctors' offices and hospitals and they are filled to capacity. Pharmacies are constantly busy filling thousands of prescriptions daily. Why? We have become an unhealthy "sick" nation. TV ads are dominated by prescription medication ads. Charles Stanley points out that we are a nation that is the richest in healthcare services and information, yet we are abusing, misusing and neglecting our bodies.[47] Americans tend to take better care of their cars than their bodies.

God first created Adam from the dust of the earth.

And the LORD God formed man of the dust of the ground, and breathed into his nostrils the breath of life; and man became a living soul.

Genesis 2:7

This "dust" of the earth contained all the minerals assimilated by plant life. We are formed of the same organic chemicals as plants. From the soil come the chemical elements such as carbon, hydrogen, and oxygen. The only chemical difference between soil and human beings is that the chemical elements in our bodies are structured in a more highly-evolved order than they are when found in the topsoil of the planet.[20] However, we cannot assimilate or metabolize chemical elements from the soil, we must obtain them from the animals and plants.

We were created by God with a magnificent physical body comprised of bones, muscles, blood, skin, etc., and a mind with emotions, free-will, soul, and a spirit. Each of these physical attributes requires a consistent, balanced intake of physical nutrients to function effectively. Much like we understand and rely upon the law of physics for our understanding of the world, we have the laws of God to govern our understanding of our bodies and our health, but how fortunate are we that God's law is written by His own finger upon every nerve, every muscle, every bone, and every cell that has been entrusted to us. Our bodies belong to God and we have a responsibility to take care of it as evidenced in Ephesians 2:10 and 1 Corinthians 6:19-20:

For we are his workmanship, created in Christ Jesus for good works, which God prepared beforehand that we should walk in them.

Ephesians 2:10

Or do you not know that your body is the temple of the Holy Spirit who is in you, whom you have of God, and you are not your own? For you were bought with a price; therefore glorify God in your body, and in your spirit, which are God's.

1 Corinthians 6:19-20

It is my belief that God is greatly dishonored when we mistreat our bodies and, "He will not work a miracle to counteract perverse violations of the laws of life and health."[53] Arthur Pink states it ever so bluntly, "The fact is that those who neglect the laws of health are carried away by disease, notwithstanding God's mercy." This is never more evident in those that continue to eat highly acidic foods of high protein, highly rancid fats and no vegetables and wonder why they get kidney stones. "Unspeakably solemn is it to see so many abusing this Divine perfection. They continue to despise God's authority, trample upon His laws, continue in sin, and yet presume upon His mercy."[30]

"You can't keep violating God's laws of life and health by misuse, abuse and neglecting your body and then ask God to heal you, so that you can then continue to misuse, abuse and neglect your body," as Charles Stanley so aptly states.[47] Could it be personal abuse when people ask for prayer for a disease that they brought upon themselves through abuse and neglect?

Staying healthy is about maintaining proper equilibrium, or homeostasis, between body, mind, and spirit. We are living in an extremely toxic and hostile world today. In order to keep our lives in balance and protect ourselves and our families from unnecessary health issues in the future, we should consider biblical principles to guard against the onslaughts and temptations that affect us. This is not about a rigid set of rules, but rather about faithfulness to healthy lifestyles.

2

✳ ✳ ✳ ✳ ✳ ✳

The Historical Evidence

Remember your leaders, those who spoke the word of God to you;
consider the outcome of their way of life and imitate their faith.

Hebrews 13:7

In Hebrews 13:7, we are reminded to remember our former leaders who spoke the word of God. A pattern of faith was set long ago for us to follow. As Jordan Rubin of *The Maker's Diet* states, "Regardless of your religious preference, any honest student of the Scriptures must admit that the wisdom of the Bible extends far beyond the spiritual issues to encompass every area of life —including dietary, hygienic, and moral guidelines."[39]

> *And God said, Behold, I have given you every herb bearing seed,*
> *which is upon the face of all the earth, and every tree, in the*
> *which is the fruit of a tree yielding seed; to you it shall be for*
> *food.*
>
> Genesis 1:29

In Genesis a pure vegetarian diet of plants is outlined. Genesis 1:29 was God's original diet for mankind—a plant-based diet of primarily raw foods. It wasn't until after the fall, when Adam disobeyed God and had to slay an animal for coverings, that animals were used as food. Prior to this, there was no express permission to slaughter animals for food.

The Old Testament gave God's people moral laws, and at the same time God gave His dietary guidelines. While the moral guidelines preserved spiritual purity, social order, family stability and community prosperity, the dietary guidelines preserved their physical health.[39] The dietary laws, or guidelines, were given by a loving God not to restrict His people, but to save His people from physical harm long before scientific principles of hygiene, viral or bacterial transmission were understood. [39]

Let now a little water be fetched, and wash your feet, and rest yourselves under the tree.

Genesis 18:4 (ASV)

So they shall wash their hands and their feet that they die not: and it shall be a statute for ever to them, even to him and to his seed throughout their generations.

Exodus 30:21 (ASV)

Even though some for ceremonial purposes, the above examples are a couple of examples that show how God's law taught His people the importance of hygiene.

Let's look at another example through the life of Daniel, one who was considered a wise leader in Daniel 1:8-16. Daniel became a vegetarian while in captivity. Symbolic language is used to illustrate faithful religious practices as a means of triumph over enemies and to instill moral lessons. He would not eat the king's delicacies. He knew there was something wrong with the king's food and didn't want to defile himself by eating the meat that had not been slain according to Mosaic Law.

Daniel preferred to eat vegetables and water. In the end, he faired healthier and stronger by eating the vegetables and water than those who ate the meat that was offered to a pagan god. This was wise on Daniel's part and is applicable for us today; not that we are to be under the law but that we consider and choose wisely what we eat. Meat offered to idols in our culture is not so much an issue today as it was in Daniel's time. Scripture warns:

*But some, through being hitherto accustomed to idols, eat food
as really offered to an idol; and their conscience, being weak, is
defiled. Food will not commend us to God. We are no worse off if
we do not eat, and no better off if we do. Only take care lest this
liberty of yours somehow become a stumbling block to the weak.*
1 Corinthians 8:7b-9 (RSV)

We can eat what we want, however, we are joined to Christ's church and
as owner of these bodies we have the responsibility to find out what is and
what is not good for our body. God's grace does not give us permission
to engage in harmful behavior even though something, such as food, is
available to us.

All things are lawful for me, but all things are not helpful.
1 Corinthians 6:12

We are admonished to not flaunt our liberty to others who may be weak.
One would no more intentionally drink wine in front of an alcoholic
anymore than one would consider eating a large serving of cake and ice
cream in front of a diabetic, or serving bread to someone who has Celiac
disease.

There are many scriptural references in the Bible where the people
neglected the word of God and strayed or used their Christian freedom
to justify their sin. While in Corinth, in 1 Corinthians 8, Paul taught the
principle that whatever we do, including putting food in our mouths, we
should ask, "Is this helpful to me?" And, "By doing this thing, or eating
this food, will it enslave me?" There were always consequences when we
do or eat something that is not healthy for us.

In Psalms 38:3-18, David laments the excruciating experience of
his illnesses and subsequent consequences of his sins. All dimensions
are mentioned in this passage; David's physical body, his mental state,
and his spirit. This passage is a profound example of sin equating with
sickness.

Today there are consequences in regard to ill-health because we have strayed from God's warnings about food and health. We cannot abuse our bodies with poor food and beverage choices or consuming poor quality food or beverages, and not have consequences..

Hippocrates, known as the Father of Medicine by historians, said in 431 B.C. "Let food by thy medicine." It was Hippocrates who also laid the cornerstone for modern medical and nutritional science. He believed that foods and natural cures not be separated from health care.[20] Bernard Jensen in his book, *Foods That Heal* says that Hippocrates even warned, "There are some who refuse to follow standards of right living, so they lose their health."[20]

God told the ancient nation of Israel that it could avoid the curse of disease if it obeyed His commandments and statues in Exodus 15:26.

> *And said, "If you diligently heed the voice of the Lord your God, and do what is right in His sight, give ear to His commandments and keep all His statutes, I will put none of the diseases on you, which I have brought on the Egyptians. For I am the Lord who heals you."*
>
> Exodus 15:26

None of these diseases! What an incredible promise! The people in Exodus, the nation of Israel, carefully restricted unclean meats and consumed foods rich in nutrients and lived a lifestyle that kept them free from illnesses and plagues throughout history, and they were healthier (free from the plague) than their neighbors who lived in surrounding regions.[39] Can this still be pertinent to us today? Medical science is still discovering how obedience to the ancient prescriptions saved primitive Hebrews from the scourges of epidemic plagues. Take Leprosy. Following the precepts laid down in Leviticus 13:46, the church undertook the task of segregating and excluding from the community those with the disease. Quarantine is still practiced today to control the spread of infectious diseases.

Through the religious leaders of the day, Israel was taught not to eat unclean animals. Leviticus 11:1-47, the book of the law, conveys warning of eating animals with divided hooves and those chewing cud, but also warns to avoid pig, certain species of sea creatures, winged insects, rodents, lizards, camel, and dead animals. Instead it advises to eat beef, lamb, wild game, fish, and certain fowl. Although many believe we do not now live under that law, but grace, the principle of not eating such things as rodents, lizards, and camel is applicable to today due to health reasons such as rabies and microbial organisms that these animals carry. God, the creator of all things, knew then and still knows what is healthy and unhealthy for our bodies. Many of these animals still carry disease causing organisms that are detrimental to our health. Some examples would be tularemia and trichinosis from pigs, bears, dogs, and horses. Lobsters and crayfish are scavengers that feed on dead organisms that can transmit disease. Clams and oysters concentrate viruses that cause hepatitis and paralytic or neurotoxic shellfish poisoning, as well as liver fluke infections.[55]

Hebrews 13:9-11 tells us that sacrificed foods are useless. According to Barnes' notes on Bible passages, "It is better to have the heart established with grace, or with the principles of pure religion, than with the most accurate knowledge of the rules of distinguishing the clean from the unclean among the various articles of food. Many such rules were found in the Law of Moses, and many more had been added by the refinements of Jewish rulers and by tradition. To distinguish and remember all these, required no small amount of knowledge, and the Jewish teachers, doubtless, prided themselves much on it. Paul says that it would be much better to have the principles of grace in the heart than all this knowledge; to have the mind settled on the great truths of religion than to be able to make the most accurate and learned distinctions in this matter." Now days we don't live by foods sacrificed or through rituals, we live by grace.

Although not part of our current culture, Acts 15:29 teaches us to not eat animals offered to idols, from blood, or strangled, for if we do abstain from these meats that were offered to idols, we will do well. Again, God's wisdom always prevails and He knows what is best for us.

Everything from scripture was written for a purpose to learn from and the principles are applicable to us today. If scriptures warn us to not eat the blood of animals, there was a reason for this; possibly a health reason.

From 100 to 6000 or more years ago, God's people have reaped what they sowed. They planted a vegetable or fruit seed and that grew to be whatever seed was planted and they ate of their harvest. In contrast, we are now reaping what we have been sowing in the recent one hundred years. In the last fifty years, the food we have eaten has come to us radically different than several thousand years ago. Our food, (the seeds sown), is now grown with more hormones, antibiotics, and chemicals, and is processed, packaged, and transported greater distances than ever before. "Our animals are slaughtered with overwhelming sadistic cruelty," declares author Kathy Freston.[13] And we are now reaping what we have sown as evidenced by this and other staggering statistics to follow.

Continuing to look at history we see a change in health conditions from pre-1900 compared to today's conditions. The prominent diseases of the Old Testament were "external" diseases such as skin disease, blindness, lameness, paralysis, fevers, infections, and mental illness.[24] Internal diseases were dysentery, intestinal worms, hemorrhages, dropsy, and plagues.[56a] According to Garth Ludwig, the main reason for disease in New Testament times was due in large part to satanic activity, and that those who were blind, lame, pain, or demon possessed were the works of "an enemy whose goal was to frustrate and destroy God's handiwork."[24] New diseases mentioned in the New Testament, which did not appear in the Old Testament, were edema, bleeding, worms, fever, and back deformities. Many diseases were associated with poverty—crowded, unsanitary living conditions, lack of clean water, failure to properly dispose of human waste, and lack of protection against disease bearing insects.[55]

According to the research of Dr. William Kneebone, DC, the top causes of death pre-1900 were: war, infections, leprosy, plagues, TB, and cholera.[21] Kneebone compares this to the top five causes of death post-1900 as: heart disease, cancer, medical drugs, hospital infections, and accidents.[21] According to Douglas S. Winnail, infectious diseases in the early 1900's were the leading cause of suffering and death in America and Europe. Even with the introduction of antibiotics, new infectious diseases have been emerging. Comparing these causes with the top ten prevalent diseases of the 1990's in the United States, according to the American Heart Association in 1998 and the Center for Disease Control in 2009, we as a nation are now are experiencing:

1998 American Heart Association	2009 CDC Diseases
1. Obesity	Heart Disease
2. Diabetes	Cancer
3. Hypertension	Respiratory Tract
4. Heart Attacks/Heart Disease	Stroke
5. Diverticulitis	Accidents
6. Cancer	Alzheimer's
7. Peptic Ulcer	Diabetes
8. Hiatal Hernia	Influenza
9. Appendicitis	Nephritis
10. Gallstones	Suicide

2016 Top World Diseases

Auto-immune
Heart Disease– 380,000 deaths in U.S. yearly
Stroke– 6.7 million affected
COPD– 6.4 million
Respiratory infections– 3.1 million
Lung Cancer– 1.6 million
Diarrheal diseases– 1.5 million
Diabetes– 1.5 million
Pre-term birth complications– 1.1 million
TB– 900,000 deaths
Malaria– 300-500 million contract
Intestinal worms––––– plague half of the human race

Alzheimer's– 5.4 million Americans

Disease was common in biblical times and will continue to be present due to the fall of Adam. However, the diseases listed above as referenced by Jordan Rubin in his book, *The Maker's Diet*, are the result of LIFESTYLE and DIET.[39] Most of these illnesses were not found in "primitive societies" of the past that consumed "primitive" (Bible-like) diets, or in third world countries today. Diet appears to be a foundational factor of disease along with: twenty percent genetics, toxins, emotional / mental stressors, lifestyle factors and cultural trends. Thirty-six percent of women and thirty-three percent of men today are overweight. One third of the diet today is junk food, comments Charles Stanley.[47]

In addition to these ten diseases, it is important to know that just within the late 1990's and early 2000; there has been an influx of new top diseases. According to Len Horowitz, these were named "emerging" diseases. They include Flesh Eating Bacteria, MRSA, Hanta Virus, Mad Cow, Bird Flu, Swine Flu, and others. More information can be read about these in Dr. Len Horowitz's book called, *Emerging Viruses: AIDS & Ebola, Nature, Accident, or Intentional.*

"This is the generation of children that will not outlive their parents." (NEJM 2005)

3

......

How Did We Get Out of Balance?

First of all, we need to ask, "What is health?" **Health** is not just the absence of disease or symptoms. Symptoms can be suppressed, masked, compensated, or accepted as normal. It is generally assumed that if one never catches a cold or flu and has no diagnosed disease that they are healthy. Not true. *True health* exhibits homeostasis—without the use of drugs, energy, and peace under stress, and seamless adaptation to physical or emotional onslaught. **Disease** is dis-"ease" or "disorder" because it wrecks human order. It is an altered biological and physiological functioning of the body due to an attack of pathogens or other malfunctions which result in damage to cells, tissues, or organs.[22] Some argue that disease is an idea or philosophy and needs a medical diagnosis in order to suppress it.

Since "the Fall" there were explicit and distinct diseases like Polio, Leprosy, Stroke, fractures and others. Over time behaviors like gambling, alcoholism, and rebelliousness were added in the classification of diseases. Now the term is used to describe a multitude of not just physiological problems, but also emotions, and behaviors.

Looking at the previous page of statistics, how did we get so "disordered?" Let's look back at history again. God laid down instructions years ago and made a promise. Leprosy was brought under control because of obedience. During the 18th century, intestinal diseases such as cholera, dysentery, and typhoid killed millions of lives. Why? Human waste. And again, God set into place thousands of years ago in order for us to avoid disease. We see in Deuteronomy 23:12-13, how to dispose properly of human waste. "Designate a place outside of camp....."

Leviticus in Chapter 15 describes that body fluids can be a vehicle for transmitting disease. We were given this warning centuries ago. These "laws" were not just ceremonial rituals, rather a set of guidelines for preventing disease. Even today, the medical establishment reminds us in public restrooms to wash hands after use.

Heredity, poor food quality, deception, sin (or disobedience to God), as well as from poor immune dysfunction are many of the reasons we have gotten out of balance. Physical health depends on the efficient functioning of the immune system.[24] What is our immune system? In simplistic terms, our immune system consists of blood, plasma, and lymph. Blood regulates body fluid volume and temperature, facilitates bodily processes like homeostasis and pH, transports and delivers oxygen and nourishment, removes wastes, transports hormones and enzymes. Blood contains platelets, red blood cells and white blood cells. White blood cells contain neutrophils, basophils and eosinophils, and are responsible for the body's defense against foreign substances. Plasma is a liquid consisting of 90% water, proteins, and hormones. Lymph transports fluids, carries away excess fluid from interstitial spaces in tissues and returns it to the bloodstream, absorbs digested fats and transports them to venous circulation, launches attacks against foreign particles such as bacteria or viruses. It is our first line of defense against invading microorganisms. It flows through filtration and collection points called nodes. These filter and destroy foreign substances. For lymph to flow it depends on contraction of smooth muscle and deep breathing. If there is an obstruction in the lymphatic system through parasites, cancer, excess wastes, poor muscle contraction, shallow breathing, node removal, then immunity can be compromised, drainage is hampered, and fluids accumulate leading to edema.

Satan will use whatever weakness he can to bring us down, confuse us and tempt us to stray from what God intended as best for us. No one argues that Typhoid fever is a disease, but Spring fever or Cabin fever, some are now arguing, are diseases and in need of medication.

Genesis 3:14 teaches us about the consequences of disobedience, loss of communion with God, nature, removal of humans from paradise to the ordinary world. There is God's way and there is man's way; truth and conjecture. We want to achieve things our own way without God, with desires for comfort. We are not satisfied with what we are given. Adam and Eve had it all; the best purest, clean, wholesome, nutritious food, peace, and joy; yet it wasn't enough. They wanted more and were deceived by Satan into thinking that more was better. It was the exaltation of self, fueled by pride which became the beginning of the fall. Times have not changed. People still are driven by desires for comfort rather than what is best. The Serpent continues to "prowl around like a lion seeking those to whom he would devour." 1 Peter 5:8. This can also be applied to our health.

There are many accounts of how people are ruining their health by destructive behavior such as with smoking, alcohol, drug, and food addictions. But, it is not just these behaviors that are ruining people's health. Drugs, whether on the street or at the pharmacy or used in order to help us face life, if we put enough of these substances or use the wrong medications, we desecrate the temple of the Living God, states Charles Stanley.[47] Eating unhealthy foods, or overeating healthy foods, I believe, also desecrates the temple, and will eventually have dire consequences. Victor Rocine in1930 stated, "If we eat wrongly, no doctor can cure us; if we eat rightly no doctor is needed."[20] I believe this is wisdom that is applicable today.

Besides our own choices in food, consider America's failing health records due in part from the U.S. government that subsidizes the very crops identified as being the most harmful to human health: corn, wheat, soy.

Garth Ludwig states, "It is significant that sickness, more than any other of life's misfortunes, stimulates people to seek spiritual solutions for their suffering."[24] We need to use discretion with our choices that could lead to desecrating the temple of the Holy Spirit, rather than ignoring God's physical principles and then seek prayer to be healed of sickness.

How else have we gotten veraciously out of balance? Below is my recipe for how we consume a toxic soup in daily life. Although an exaggeration, it points to how easy it is to be exposed to toxins if we are not watchful and diligent.

Recipe for Toxic Soup

Ingredients:

½ inch of fluoride toothpaste

3 scoops of Listerine mouth wash

1 ounce of Irish Spring soap

1 application of Speed Stick antiperspirant/deodorant

1 tablespoon of non-organic body lotion

6 tablets of prescription medications

2 tablets of antibiotics

2 sprays of air deodorizer

7 cups of tap water

10 pounds of Genetically Modified corn, wheat, and soy in our meals

1 nonorganic potato fried in Teflon skillet, followed by 2 nonorganic eggs, 1 doughnut and coffee for breakfast, or 1 bagel made with white flour containing oxidizing agents, with 16 ounces of Mocha Latte coffee

1 cup coffee with artificial sweetener

5 inhalations of carbon monoxide

2 inhalations of diesel fuel

3 inhalations of cigarette smoke

½ gallon of pesticide spray

3 doses of window cleaner

20 mile dash of jogging along a busy street (inhaling toxic fumes from auto exhaust and cadmium from tires)

3 rounds of 100 push-ups, 200 sit ups, 200 pull ups (over exertion)

500 calories daily or 6000 calories daily

6 ounce steak from cows fed growth hormones, antibiotics, and tranquilizers, and 1 large potato for lunch or dinner

5 ounces of nonorganic chicken raised with antibiotics and hormones

2 cups French fries, 64 oz. diet soda, 6 Oreo cookies with 2 cups non-fat milk for snack

1 Lunchable

Consume 3-4 days of left-overs weekly

1 TV dinner, and salad with store bought dressing loaded with a collection of preservatives, colorings, flavorings, and artificial sweeteners with a dinner roll and margarine containing trans fats

Eat out at fast food restaurants two to three times a week

Add 6-7 servings of food additives, flavorings, colors, preservatives

Spend 60 minutes on a cell phone and 6 hours on a computer

Travel overseas frequently

Stir in 96+ vaccines over a lifetime

Instructions:

1. Mix all ingredients together day after day, month after month, year after year.
2. Add genetic disorders stemming from a relative.
3. Stir in emotional trauma.
4. Continue with negative self-talk.
5. Insert 2 amalgam fillings in teeth.
6. Consume on a daily basis. Enjoy a life filled with fatigue, drowsiness, headaches, rashes, nausea, joint pain, ringing in the ears, swollen glands, hormonal imbalances, hair loss, difficulty concentrating, memory loss, dizziness, edema, irritability, chronic degenerative disease, and overall system degeneration.

How we Acquire Dis-ease (Figure 1)

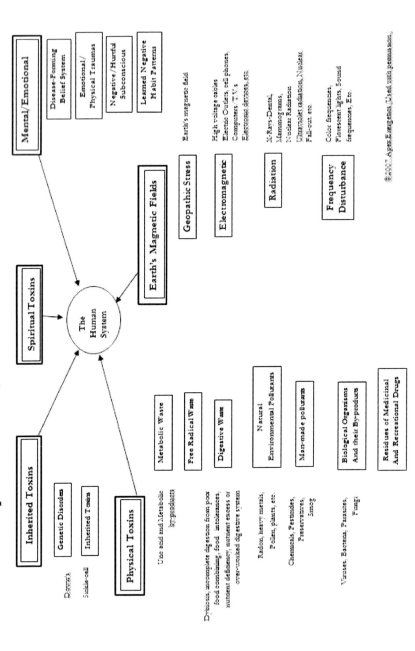

Mental/Emotional
- Disease-Forming Belief System
- Emotional/ Physical Traumas
- Negative/Hurtful Subconscious
- Learned Negative Habit Patterns

Spiritual Toxins

Inherited Toxins
- Genetic Disorders
- Inherited Toxins

Down's

Sickle-cell

Physical Toxins

The Human System

Earth's Magnetic Fields

Geopathic Stress — Earth's magnetic field

Electromagnetic — High voltage cables, Electric Outlets, cell phones, Computers, T.V.'s Electronic devices, etc.

Radiation — X-Rays-Dental, Mammograms, Nuclear Radiation Ultraviolet radiation, Nuclear Fall-out, etc.

Frequency Disturbance — Color frequencies, Fluorescent lights, Sound frequencies, Etc.

- Metabolic Waste
- Free Radical Waste
- Digestive Waste — Uric acid and Metabolic by-products

Dysbiosis, incomplete digestion from poor food combining, food intolerances, nutrient deficiency, nutrient excess or over-worked digestive system

- Natural Environmental Pollutants — Radon, heavy metals, Pollen, plants, etc.
- Man-made pollutants — Chemicals, Pesticides, Preservatives, Smog
- Biological Organisms And their By-products — Viruses, Bacteria, Parasites, Fungi
- Residues of Medicinal And Recreational Drugs

©2007 Apex Energetics (Used with permission)

Figure one graphically displays further ways we have become out of balance or disordered. The human body with all its checks and balances can only handle so many onslaughts. There are a number of factors to take into consideration contributing to disorder and disease. All these factors, broken down into these five categories, bombard the human system.

First, **inherited toxins** are blamed for almost anything now days when in actuality there is a relatively small percentage of diseases that are inherited based on chromosome mutation. There is an element of truth here dating back over 2000 years ago.

Times have not changed. More children are being born with diseases some believed to be impossible in newborns. Scientists are now finding babies born with over 200 chemicals in umbilical cord blood as pointed out in *Scientific American* in 2009. This means their disease is inherited. If generation after generation has smoked, taken recreational drugs, drank alcohol, emotionally abusive, lived on "junk food," or were exposed to toxins knowingly or unknowingly, or have transgressed from God's physical or moral laws, the damage will be passed down through generations. A person's actions still determines whether or not he/she succumbs to disease. Alcoholism is no more inherited than influenza!

> *'The Lord is slow to anger and abounding in steadfast love, forgiving iniquity and transgression, but he will by no means clear the guilty, visiting the iniquity of the fathers on the children, to the third and the fourth generation.'*
> Numbers 14:18 (ESV)

Numbers 14:18 is an example of generational cycles of sin. Unless someone in the family line makes a conscientious effort to change patterns of behavior or practices, that behavior or practice will be passed from parent to child. This is called sowing and reaping. However, the sins of parents are not always passed down in ill health. An example of this is in the book of John.

And His disciples asked Him, saying, "Rabbi, who sinned, this

man or his parents, that he should be born blind?" Jesus answered,
"[It was] neither [that] this man sinned, nor his parents; but [it
was] in order that the works of God might be displayed in him.

John 9:2-3 (NAS)

Here Jesus denies that the illness was due to sin passed down. And even
if the illnesses were due to sin, Jesus many times forgave the sins of those
whom He healed.[24]

Second, **spiritual toxins** in the realm of spiritual warfare, is a factor
that has been around since the fall of Adam and Eve. We have seen
this in persecutions in the name of religious freedom. The Apostle Paul
tells us to put on our spiritual armor because our battle in this world is
a "spiritual" one. This warfare involves the deception and power of the
devil, as opposed to a human battle. The battlefield also takes place in the
mind of believers. We wrestle, or strive and struggle in our minds against
world systems, the flesh or the carnal nature. The mind encompasses our
thoughts (imagination, reasoning, and intellect) as well as our emotions
and will. This can be a contributing factor in mental and emotional stress.

Third, **mental/emotional toxins** from negative self-talk, negative or
emotional abuse, physical abuse, or even learned negative habit patterns.
"Eating fat will make me fat," "I have to count calories," "I don't have
any disease, so my weight is fine," "I'm just not good enough," "I can't
do this," "I'm worthless," "I can't stand the way I look," "There is no
hope for me," "There is nothing to be happy about," are all examples of
emotional toxins, are counter-productive and when not kept in check
can grow into emotional toxic burdens on the body. We see this warning
for negative self-talk in Proverbs 23 below.

For as he thinks in his heart, so is he.

Proverbs 23:7

For further reading on controlling toxic emotions, I recommend the
book, *Who Switched off my Brain?* by Caroline Leaf, PhD.

Fourth, **physical toxins**, I believe, are the main reason we acquire disease. Our bodies circulate metabolic waste daily. If our elimination channels are blocked in any way, these metabolic by-products will accumulate in our body and will have a serious effect on our metabolism and health. Our metabolism can also be damaged by excessive exercising and inappropriate yo-yo dieting. Digestive wastes come from food, food intolerances, poor food combining, and nutrient deficiencies as well as nutrient excesses, or poor nutrition, overworked digestive systems, and the Standard American Diet (SAD) which is explained further later. This sets the stage for inflammatory reactions and the cycle of more food intolerances and digestive issues such as dysbiosis, incomplete digestion, malabsorption, an overworked digestive system and diseases such as Crohn's Disease, irritable bowel syndrome, and diverticulitis.

One common mistake in food customs is to eat too much too frequently, taking the next meal before the previous one has been assimilated. Some dieticians are telling peole to eat every 2-3 hours. This overworks the digestive organs.[20] Just as harmful to the digestive tract is to space meals too far apart depleting energy stores and taxing the pancreas.

Victor Rocine during the 1930's, proposed that nutrient deficiency or excess of any of the primary chemical elements (vitamins and minerals and other chemical compounds from food) was at the root of most human disease, maladies, and mental problems, and encouraged that we should eat food the way God manufactures it for us.[20] And how might we, as a nation with abundance of food, become nutrient deficient?

Fifth, **natural and environmental pollutants** come from radon, heavy metals, chromium from car tires, paints, inks, textiles, and wood preservatives, pollen, and "acid rain." Another environmental pollutant not commonly thought about is aflatoxins. These are mycotoxins that come from fungus or mold and are quite toxic to humans and animals due to the havoc they wreck on the liver and gastrointestinal tract. These molds are found in unsuspecting places such as contaminated grains, (before harvest or due to long storage), poor soil, milk from animals fed contaminated feed, and berries. One moldy berry in a basket contaminates the entire basket. Even peanut butter is susceptible to this toxin.

Man-made pollutants are chemicals in drugs, pesticides, fertilizers, preservatives, cosmetics, personal care products, medications, processed foods, smog from vehicle emissions, and phthalates from plastics. Plastics are a modern day invention and have shown in studies to cause infertility and contribute to estrogen excess.[37] Bisphenol A (BPA) is a chemical found in plastics; especially the flimsy ones containing bottled water. One study found that low levels — two parts per billion — of BPA disrupts the endocrine systems of laboratory animals causing birth defects.[12] Another study found BPA can lead to learning disabilities in children and neurodegenerative diseases in adults.[12] Studies in rats have shown estrogenic chemical exposures (phthalates) caused changes in the mammary and pituitary glands.[37] Consider how often in a day you use plastics from water bottles, baby bottles, food wrappers, food storage, dry cleaning covers, plastic tablecloths, plastic bags, etc.

Another study on Bisphenol A showed early puberty in female rats and reduced fertility.[37] These and many others studies confirm why I believe we are seeing many more young girls with developed mammary glands and early puberty due to the amount of plastics and pesticides to which they and their mothers have been exposed. Fitzgerald reveals that twelve percent of the United States reproductive population now experiences infertility and that rate is rising overall, particularly among women under twenty-five years of age.[12] As I outlined earlier in my Recipe for Toxic Soup, countless other common sources of toxins come from the following non-organic products:

Beauty products — lotions, creams, soaps, make-up, nail polish, lipstick, body lotion

Personal care products — shampoo, conditioner, hair dyes, toothpaste, shave cream, sunscreen, scented candles, scented household products, feminine products, deodorant, mouthwash

Household cleaners — windows, kitchen, bath/shower, toilet bowl, carpets, laundry soap, dryer sheets

Prescription/OTC drugs — antacids, headache remedies, colds/cough, flu remedies, allergy remedies

Insect Repellants — sprays, lotions, gels, candles

Not only with personal care and beauty products, household and over-the-counter drugs, but the air we breathe, water we drink, food we eat, and other choices in which the products we use compromises the quality of our health and taxes the body beyond its natural capabilities of detoxification. It is the combined action of these toxins that creates a toxic soup effect that can weaken the immune system. Added to the toxic soup are biological organisms that come from viruses, bacteria, parasites, and fungi.

In addition, **thermal stress** is another factor in ill health. Hippocrates was aware that climates (weather, heat, coldness, dampness, dryness) have an effect on our health.[20] Exiting a very warm indoor environment into a very cold outside environment leads to thermal stress on the body. The opposite is true as well. This is why it is important to dress appropriately for the weather. Our bodies were not designed to adapt to such extreme temperature changes.

The next category of how we acquire disease is from **external Energy field disturbances**. Never before in the history of the world have we seen the damages from external energy fields as we are experiencing today. With high voltage cables, transformers, computers, high definition TV, and other electronic devices, X-rays, cell phones, Wi-Fi, microwaves, and nuclear radiation, our bodies are not designed to withstand the frequency output of these devices. Currently, the United States has 264 million wireless subscribers relying on cell towers and antennas. We don't even have to own a cell phone anymore to be bombarded with Radio Frequencies. Sherrill Sellman, ND documented that there has been an increase in brain tumors, neurological impairment, learning disabilities, hormone disruption, compromised immunity and cancers. Information carrying radio waves is a frequency that never existed before in nature, so our bodies perceive this as foreign and toxic to our cells; ultimately resulting in energy depleted weakened immune system; which in turn becomes more vulnerable to environmental toxins. According to Dr. Vini Khurana, a neurosurgeon, on a CBS *60 Minutes* episode in 2009, he predicts that there will be an explosion of brain tumors and other health issues due to the now prolonged use of cell phones. Although the media would have us believe that cell phones do not "cause" brain tumors, there is plenty of research to substantiate that EMF's (Electromagnetic Frequencies) promote cancer and other biological and energetic disturbances.

Next, how we got out of balance is through **deception**. Cultural pressures, perception, media ads, and food politics are some of the areas we can be deceived. According to Fitzgerald, food additives may be labeled "flavorings," or "natural," while chemicals in personal-care products might be labeled "fragrances." Pesticide ingredients are disguised under the term "inert."[12] Vitamins are now added to water and some soft drinks in an attempt to deceive the unaware that the product is healthy. Health claims on packaged foods such as "zero trans fats" or "contains whole wheat" creates an impression that a product is healthy when in fact it is false and far from being healthy. It is still packaged and usually loaded with excess salt and sugars. Processed food companies sell vegetable soup so cheaply because they load them with "high-glycemic" carbohydrates like rice, potatoes, and pasta that cost virtually nothing. Then they add inexpensive ingredients like corn, sugar, and maybe some rancid and GMO oils like cottonseed oil. Added to this are the highly cooked vegetables. For less than $2 you can get a high carb, high calorie soup that provides essentially no health benefits. But it appears healthy to the unsuspecting person because there are vegetables in the soup. Do these common practices sound like deception?

Biblically, there are many warnings about deception in the Old and New Testaments. It all started in the Garden of Eden when Eve was deceived by the serpent. Spiritual fall came to Eve through Satan in the form of a certain food.

> *And the Lord God said unto the woman, "What is this that you have done?" And the woman said, "The serpent beguiled me, and I did eat."*
>
> Genesis 3:13

> *When you sit down to eat with a ruler, consider carefully what is*

before you; And put a knife to your throat, if you are a man given to appetite. Do not desire his delicacies, for they are deceptive food.

Proverbs 23:1-3

Even though we have to look at Proverbs in context, the warning above to not give in to strong appetite and to be wary of deception is still applicable. The consequence of overindulgence and nutrient excess has become a national epidemic. Deception today still comes from Satan in numerous ways, and he continues to use food to debilitate, distract, and destroy our bodies.

Consider the deception in the United States meat industry ads. The commercials show pictures of happy cows and clucky chickens frolicking in fields, nestling in cozy straw beds in bright red barns. The reality is far removed from this picture and looks more like barbaric war zones generated from greedy profiteers capitalizing on your appetites for meat. For further information on the meat industry, view the documentary, *Food Inc.*

Consider that Nestle bought out Jenny Craig. Is there a conflict of interest here? Or, consider the snake oil salesmen of the nineteenth century who sold "special secret ingredients" in their tonics that promised cures for every ailment imaginable. The tonic was questionable, and the snake oil salesman, known as someone who sold fraudulent goods, didn't stay in business for very long. The primary focus, however, was deception through using accomplices in the audience to proclaim the benefits of the preparation.[67a]

At one time I had attended a medical appointment with my husband at a local medical facility. I noticed a new sign for "refreshments" which had replaced an optometrist's office. It caught my curiosity so I walked into this little room and to my shock saw several machines lining two of the walls selling soft drinks, chips, candy bars, cookies, coffee, and other sugar laden and refined carbohydrate food stuff. I stood there scratching my head wondering, "What were they thinking?" "This is a medical facility for crying out loud." "People come here because they are sick." Diabetes and obesity are the number one health problem in America and here is a medical facility perpetuating the epidemic of two of the most prominent health disorders. Is there a conflict of interest here? Is there deception here? Is revenue more important than the health of patients? It took years to finally get vending machines out of public schools. Now children can get their junk food fix by visiting their doctor.

As Randall Fitzgerald points out, today's chemical, drug, and food industries create equivalent deception. Each of these industries uses trade secrecy laws designed to protect their ingredients from imitation by competitors as a way to hide their special chemical ingredients from the public. Although these laws protect the industry, the deception is in denying the public an opportunity to assess the complete list of chemicals and their potential risks and safety for the products purchased.[12]

What we perceive in advertisements can feel like reality and also what we value. If we perceive that McDonald's food is not harmful that is reality for us and we value eating there, regardless of the fact that the food there could be harmful to our body no matter how cute and effective the marketing is. And Satan can do that quite effectively today through marketing. Take a look at most ads. What are these ads appealing to? And to whom are they appealing? The last twenty-five years we've seen an explosion with marketers targeting children to advertise their products. They lure and appeal to parents' emotional guilt for not spending enough time with their children, and, in turn, the parents spend money on them from fast food restaurants' "Happy Meals" toys, video games, to cell phones.[43]

Schlosser even argues that schoolchildren are now becoming a captive audience for marketers as students look at ads in the classroom setting. America's schools currently loom as a potential gold mine for companies in search of young customers.[43] I remember vividly a conversation I had with the child nutrition director of one school district about changing the menu items to more nutritious healthy choices. (This was long before Jamie Oliver began his campaign with school lunches.) Her response stunned me. "Well, we would lose revenue." I cautiously replied, "So what you are telling me is that your department making money is more important than the children's health?" Her reply.......... "Yes." One way the school lunch problem can be changed at this point is for parents to make demands with their local school board for healthier whole foods and eliminate processed foods, or send their child to school with a lunch prepared at home.

Let no one deceive you with empty words, for because of these things the wrath of God comes upon the sons of disobedience.

Ephesians 5:6

Paul, in Ephesians 5:6, was admonishing to not get caught up in deception from others. Cultural pressures, the media, and food politics are influences that can be deceptive.

A recent CBS *60 Minutes* episode with Morley Safer revealed the deception of the Food Industry and in particular that of the flavor industry. This multibillion dollar industry creates chemical flavorings that go into food products to make them palatable and mouthwatering for the sole purpose of hooking the consumer into buying more of that product. Food companies know that flavor is what makes repeat customers. The industry's main focus is to make the taste experience of the food so pleasurable that we get "addicted" to that particular product for the industry's profit; not our health, as Safer points out in his interview. The products are not real food. Artificial flavoring is nothing more than an appalling concoction of chemicals that will trick your brain into thinking you are eating something healthy and tasty, but is loaded with toxic chemicals. The secret formula flavors are copied in a chemical lab from a real food substance and then manipulated to give the impression of the original food.[42] This is blatant deception. That strawberry or vanilla flavor in a food product purchased could have come from a beaver's backside, as Safer enlightens. This is a far cry from God's original design of food.

Another form of deception that has steered this nation to dis-order exists in the pharmaceutical field. Pharmaceutical- the Greek word is "pharmakia" which means "drugs" or to practice witchcraft or demonic activity, or sorcery.[47] We get our English word "pharmacy" from the Greek word "pharmakia" denoting medicine. It appears several times in the New Testament in Galatians 5:20, Revelation 9:21, 18:23, 21:8, and 22:15.

In each of the above passages, "pharmakia," or "drugs" is listed as a work of the flesh of man as opposed to the Spirit of God working in us. The King James Bible translators translated "pharmakia" as "witchcraft," because almost no one but witches and sorcerers used drugs 400 years ago. Drugs were most commonly used in pagan worship to hallucinate and to try to get in touch with evil spirits. Drugs now are not typically associated with hallucinogenics, but rather common place acceptance for whatever ailment. According to American Psychological Association in 2010, $16 billion dollars was spent on psychiatric medications. $11 billion on antidepressants. There is a growing and disturbing trend within the church of Christians using prescription pain killers, anti-depressants, nerve pills, and other strong prescription drugs on a regular or continuing basis. If those with health challenges wanted to they may be able to reduce or eliminate the use of the prescriptions through their own self-control or life style changes.

The Bible seems to be advising us to avoid medicines that are unnecessary; and again, be wary of deception. Look at the packaging of drugs on T.V. ads! Bright colors, catchy tunes, and medical claims for particular ailments that "hook" a person into believing that drug will cure what ails them.

A little bit about pharmaceuticals:

Our cells and body systems communicate between each other in two ways: One, by electricity through the neurons (your nervous system), and two, by hormones, peptides, neurotransmitters, steroids, and other molecules (your endocrine system). These travel between cells and systems to carry messages. They are the messengers. Each one of your 100 trillion cells has tens of thousands of receptor sites. Each receptor site has specific functions and a lock that requires a specific key. For a hormone or neuron to pass its information to a cell, it has to hold the right key. Pharmaceuticals are specifically designed to block specific receptor sites or to pass false information to certain cells in order to trick the body into giving up symptoms.[49] For example, if you have a runny nose, the prescription is designed to find the cells that give rise to that symptom and trick them into stopping. It is essentially lying to the body. And who is the author of lies? Prescription drugs lie and confuse the body's cells. This is the ultimate of deception. There is a place for medicine and God will use these for our benefit, but today, too many people are over medicated. An ancient Chinese Proverb states,

"He that takes medicine and neglects diet, wastes the time of his doctor."

Are we possibly addicting ourselves to these medications? Let's take a look at a possible progression of our "drug addicted" and over medicated society. From the time children are young, if they have an earache they are put on amoxicillin. Next, they develop thrush, a side effect from the antibiotic, so they are given another medication to help with that side effect, and so on until the next earache develops. During the school years the child can't focus or is overactive so they are put on Ritalin. By high school, the child turns to No-Doz or Monster drinks to keep themself awake. Topping this off are the myriad of 69+ doses of vaccinations a child has been given since birth up to age 18. Young mothers in their 20's to 30's are so stressed out with schedules and raising young ones, they are now put on Prozac or other antidepressants. The years between ages 30 and 60 people are realizing they can't digest their food and are plagued with heartburn or acid reflux, so are put on Zantax or Protonics. By the time retirement age and older, and person has spent their life on some sort of prescription or OTC drug and now their physiology is so damaged that they require more drugs to control cholesterol, diabetes, heart disease, and all the side effects that come with all the prescriptions, to keep them from the degenerative disease that they already have. This perpetuating cycle is the predominant picture in the culture in which Americans are currently living. Over time all these drugs dull our senses, degenerate our bodies, and can lead to other apparent or unapparent addictions. Our bodies were not equipped to handle the plethora of prescription drugs.

Today's ads, social media, and marketing gimmicks use special offers and celebrity endorsements as hooks that lure people into purchasing products. Food politics alone are involved in a vast majority of deception. Countless warnings to be wary abound in scripture. This is wisdom for today's culture of deception in the health and food industry.

In addition to the above toxins, is air pollution. Our cardiovascular and pulmonary systems support every bodily function. They operate as a perfectly choreographed team to deliver the oxygen essential for our life's functions, and disposes the deadly carbon dioxide produced by metabolic processes. God designed a perfectly healthy oxygen rich air in the beginning. It was God who breathed the first breath of air into man as we see in Genesis.

And God said, "Let there be space between the waters, to separate water from water," And so it was. God made this space to separate the waters above from the waters below. And God called the space, "sky."

Genesis 1:6-8 (NLT)

And the Lord God formed man of the dust of the ground, and breathed into his nostrils the breath of life; and man became a living being.

Genesis 2:7

The air we breathe today is not what it used to be. Air pollution is a major problem in the US both outdoors and indoors. US government rates it as the number one environmental problem. American College of Allergists blame 50% of all allergy related illnesses on indoor pollutants. EPA states that indoor air is 200 times worse than outdoor air. Most people spend over 90% of their time indoors.

Latest research has shown that the inside air quality is more hazardous than the outside air. Sometimes fresh air will prove far more beneficial to sick people than medicine. The health of the entire system depends upon the healthy action of the respiratory organs.[53]

Every cell of your body must receive a constant supply of oxygen or they will weaken and die. The air must be fresh in order to benefit the most. When we breathe stale or polluted air, the supply of oxygen is insufficient to keep the cells strong and healthy. Homes built in biblical times were open; the air was fresh and clean.

Houses built today are airtight unfortunately trapping pollutants and allergens inside (as much as 200% higher) Several of the effects produced by living in close, ill ventilated rooms are as follows: The system becomes weak and unhealthy, the circulation is depressed, the blood moves sluggishly through the system, the mind becomes depressed and gloomy, and fevers and other acute diseases are liable to be generated. How many of have experienced "Cabin Fever?" If you've ever had difficulty going to sleep, try opening a window to let fresh air circulate.

A Scientific American article stated that a baby crawling on the floor at home breathes in the equivalent of four cigarettes per day because of chemicals from the carpeting, molds, mildews, dust mites, etc. emit toxic off-gases.

Smog is composed of chemicals and other polluted matter found in the air. The three major components are ozone, particulate matter and NOx (nitrogen oxide). There are over two hundred air toxics in California that are irritants, carcinogens, or reproductive toxins. Smog is responsible for three million lost work hours each year in Southern California. There are 300 cancer deaths directly related to smog each year in California. Long term exposure can lead to fibrosis or scarring of the respiratory tissue resulting in up to 50% decreased breathing capacity.[21]

The concentration of uranium in the soil or bedrock off-gases into the air. If a building is built over an area of high concentration, the level of off-gassed radon in the house or other building from the soil can be dangerously high. It is the second leading cause of lung cancer in US. 1 in 15 houses in the US have high levels of radon. EPA estimates that between 3,000-32,000 people die annually due to radon exposure. Since 1976 there has been a 100% increase in radon exposure related health issues.[37]

There are many other air pollutants that are causing a decrease in our health, and does all this have an effect on our food? Yes! Plants take in oxygen too. Toxic air can produce toxic plants. When acidic air pollutants combine with water droplets in clouds, the water becomes acidic. This is known as "Acid Rain." When those droplets fall to the ground, the plants take up the water from the now contaminated soil. Damage due to acid rain kills plants, trees and harms animals, fish, and other wildlife. Acid rain also changes the chemistry of the water in lakes and streams, harming fish and other aquatic life. This is a minute example of the fall-out of air pollution and the domino effect it has on plants and ultimately our health.

Simple solutions for air pollution

1. Use air purifiers
2. Spend time outside on non-smog days
3. Practice deep breathing
4. Be earth friendly; recycle
5. Have plants inside the home to help oxygenate the indoor air

Looking at the staggering statistics of disease in our generation reveals how far we have strayed. In comparison to biblical times the list might include the number of fallen comrades or deaths from infections or leprosy. The statistics below just did not exist in biblical times. And the percentages are getting worse. According to the DSM (Disease and Statistics Manual), over 400 new diseases existed in 2006. Current number is 13,000, but this changes constantly. As the DSM grows, so do the number of people who are sick. Do you think there is a correlation here? Millions of dollars are spent on cancer a year, and yet the number of deaths is not decreasing.[12] The majority of these diseases are due to lifestyle and diet factors.[12]

Statistics and Disease

» $2.6 trillion is spent on health care a year and 30 percent of this is spent on unnecessary tests, procedures, medications, and hospital stays (2008 Congressional Budget Office estimate)

» The average consumption of sugar in 2 to 3 year olds is 14 teaspoons a day (*J. of Pediatrics*, Jan. 2005)

» 46% of people in Netherlands walk for transportation, 7% in USA

» The average American consumes 60 pounds of cakes, cookies, 23 gallons of ice cream, 7 pounds of potato chips, 365 servings of soda, and 756 doughnuts a year

» 10 billion land animals (35 million cattle, 100 million pigs, 300 million turkeys, about 5 billion fish, and about 9.5 billion chickens) are killed each year for food [19]

» Americans drink about 56 gallons of soda per person annually.[43]

» 2 out of 10 Americans have been diagnosed with irritable bowel syndrome

» A generation ago three-quarters of the money used to buy food in the United States was spent to prepare meals at home. Today about half of the money used to buy food is spent at restaurants—mainly fast food restaurants [43]

» 26% patients discharged from hospitals are more malnourished than when they went in. 80% of the reason they went in is due to their poor state of nutrition [8]

» A typical American now consumes approximately three hamburgers and four orders of French fries every week [43]

» 2 million people are admitted to hospital emergency rooms from drug reactions from prescriptions or over-the-counter medications

» In 2006, 1.3 million coronary angioplasty procedures were performed, 448,000 coronary bypass operations costing more than $100 billion (*"Alternative Medicine Is Mainstream."* The Wall Street Journal. 2009)

» The number one leading cause of deaths is heart disease

» Lipitor is the most prescribed drug in the world for cholesterol (Matt Ledermen, M.D. *Forks Over Knives*, 2011)

» More than 100,000 people die every year from prescription

drugs properly administered

» 250,000 iatrogenic (physician facilitated) deaths a year

» 2 billion people suffer from micronutrient deficiencies worldwide

» There is an estimated 734,000 suicide attempts in the United States annually; for every 25 attempts there is one death [54]

» Immune Statistics (U.S.)

» 73 million have chronic respiratory conditions

» 70 million adults/30 million children have arthritis

» 17 million have Type 2 diabetes a 70% increase since 1977

» 400,000 have MS

» 850,000 – 950,000 have AIDS (more than 1mil. are infected with the virus)

» CDC has counted more than 800,000 AIDS cases since 1981 and 460,000 deaths

» 2 million have ileitis and colitis

» 1960 -13% of Staph infections were resistant to penicillin. In 1997—99% (www.educate-yourself.org/ed/index.shtml, 2009)

» 250,000-300,000 Americans die per year from the top three infections (sepsis, influenza, pneumonia) (*Rising Plague*, by Brad Spellberg, M.D.)

» 170,000 Americans died of infections in 1996; a doubling in the number over the previous three decades (*Rising Plague*, by Brad Spellberg, M.D.)

» 2 cans of cola can depress white blood cell function by 92% for as long as 5 hours (*J. Archives of Surgery* 1999; 134:1229)

Cancer Statistics

» 44% increase since 1950

» 100% increase in Prostate Cancer – 1950

» Breast Cancer–1:20–1950, 1990s–1:8, now 1:7

» Melanoma cases are up 690 percent since 1950 [12]

» Prostate cancer up 286 percent since 1950 [12]

» Thyroid cancer up 258 percent since 1950 [12]
» Cancer Deaths: 1/minute, 1500/day, 10,000/week, 500,000/ year = 3 – 747s crashing/day (CDC 2009)
» United States ranks 25th in the world for number of cancer diagnosis
» World Health Organization researchers estimate that by 2020 cancer diagnosis rates will increase another 50%
» 7 million deaths from cancer; 1 million in U.S. alone. (2002 Sunlight Nutrition & Health Research) and, these statistics will be increasing yearly[12]

Obesity Statistics

» U.S. Surgeon General declared in December 2001 that American was in the midst of an epidemic of obesity that threatens the nation's health
» About 300,000 deaths a year due to complications of obesity[47]
» $240 billion is spent on health care costs annually for obesity[43]
» In 1999, 60% of adults and 13% of children in U.S. were obese. 2010, 1/3 of adults and 17% of children which equates to 78 million adults and 13 million children aged 2-19
» $40 million is spent on weight loss diets annually (Bloomberg Business Week)
» 70% of the nation is regarded as overweight. (AARP January-February 2012)

Mental Health Statistics

» 20 million American adults have anxiety disorder of some type
» Over 2 million have panic disorder
» 5 million have post traumatic stress disorder
» 4 million children have ADHD
» 2 million have bipolar disorder

Environmental Statistics

» 20,000 of the 70,000 toxic chemicals in our environment are known carcinogens
» 2 billion pounds- pesticides are sprayed on our food each year
» 9 million pounds- Antibiotics given to animal/year
» 90 billion pounds of Toxic waste dumped at 55,000 waste sites/year
» 20-25% of population has allergies (50 Million)

These statistics do not include the amounts of hormones injected into animals per year to fatten them up

Broken bones can be set, infections can be eliminated, cancer can be "cured," but no mental illness can be cured. The statistics above is depressing enough to send us running for some antidepressants! But, there are alternatives and solutions as you will see later in this book.

What were the factors leading to disease during biblical times? Inherited toxins, infections, Spiritual Warfare, and mental/emotional toxins, and as we saw earlier, or consequences of disobedience to God's commands. In biblical times, obviously, there were no electromagnetic frequencies, no radon, no heavy metals, and no man-made pollutants from factories, or medicinal and recreational drug residues with which to contend. After reading Daniel's account of not eating meat, the other men could very well have battled dysbiosis and poor digestion from the meats offered to idols, the very ones that God warned about—natural consequences.

As Debbie Williams exhorts, "To deny the effects of toxins in our body is to deny warnings given to us by health care professionals and nutritionists." "To deny the existence and influence of Satan and the toxic effect of sin for us spiritually is to deny our Lord's warnings."[54]

How Toxic Are We?

According to a report by the CDC, 116 known toxic chemicals were found in large percentages of the population.[37] The EPA has been conducting National Human Adipose Tissue Studies since 1976. The latest study reported shows that 54 chemical toxins were found in alarming levels in adipose tissue. DDT, a pesticide–banned in 1973 in US, is currently exported to South America and Mexico. We eat fruit and vegetables imported from Mexico. DDE is a very toxic by-product of DDT. DDE has been detected in 100% of all samples of raisins, spinach, beef and chili con carne. In the United States, it has been found in 93% of cheese, hamburger, hot dogs, bologna, collards, chicken, ice cream sandwiches and turkey. DDE contamination has caused disorders in animal studies of the nervous system, liver, kidney, immune system, adrenals, and sterility. It has also been associated with pancreatic cancer in humans. DDT has a half- life (the time it takes for half a given amount of a substance such as a drug to be removed from living tissue through natural biological activity) of 2-15 years.[37] It is very difficult to remove from soil or water tables and is quite toxic to aquatic invertebrates and vertebrates.

DDT is estrogen-like. 1 molecule is equal to 3,000 molecules of estrogen.[37] The problem with this is that this can add to the toxic soup of xenoestrogens in a women's body that have already been built up from estrogens consumed from soybeans, animals injected with hormones, and other foods, as well as from plastics. Sad is the fact that estrogen dominance is a leading cause in breast cancer.

DDT, PCB's and Dioxins are examples of hundreds of other toxic chemicals in our environment. Researchers are uncertain about the long term effects of all but a few of them. Add to all of this, we are exposed to 100 million times more electropollutants today than in 1950. So how toxic are we? Very toxic! All of us are walking around with some degree of toxicity.

So, how did we get out of balance? Toxins! In spite of all the toxins around us, we can overcome! It is only by His grace that we are able to survive in this toxic world. Our hope should be in Him who is in control of all things.

David Stewart, PhD, states, "When most people are sick, they don't go to church to be anointed and healed as early Christians once did.

They first go to doctors or hospitals to get a drug or OTC medication."[47] God's intent is for us to take responsibility for our own health care using the intelligence He gave us, guided by Him in prayer.

4

· · · · · ·

Eating the Worldly Way, The Standard American Diet

The Standard American Diet (SAD), the junk food diet of America and now in surrounding countries since the introduction of Fast Food restaurants, consists of:

Refined, dead, food
Stored for lengthy time periods
Overcooked food
Enzyme depleted
Processed
Trans fats-hydrogenated/partially hydrogenated,
High fat
Hormones injected in food
Antibiotics injected in food
Pesticide ridden
Additives
Preservatives
Genetically altered
Pasteurized, homogenized
Sweetened
Chemical sweeteners

This translates to:

Fast food restaurants
Packaged foods
Microwaved foods
Commercial baked goods of cupcakes, pies, cookies, cakes,
    brownies, chips, doughnuts
An enormous amount of excess fat, and sugar consumption
Refined wheat products including white bread, crackers, bagels,
    pasta, and cereals
Energy drinks, and sodas

Add to that the poor nutrient quality of the soil and plants, and we have a body that is toxic, oxidized, inflamed, and most likely lacking energy. Then by the time we are 35 or 40 years old we are walking around like an 80 year old with all kinds of ails and wondering what hit us! Or we find ourselves running around trying every remedy or supplement to cure our symptoms, or trying every diet imaginable to quickly take off the accumulated pounds. According to Robin Miller in *Kneeling at the Altar of Obesity*, "We're obsessed in this country with trying to find some reason other than our own bad eating and exercise habits to explain our ever-growing waistlines," and poor health, that I might add.

Studies show that a steady diet of junk food will bring harm. Just because that food exists does not mean we should eat it.

All things are lawful, but not all things are profitable. All things are lawful, but not all things edify.
1 Corinthians 10:23 (NASB)

According to Charles Stanley, "As food is to the body, so obedience is to the soul and spirit."[45] As Daniel, in the Old Testament, refused the King's food, he was being obedient and knew that the King's food was not profitable to his body. The King's food of today is junk food; although I am sure it has not been offered to idols. Yet most junk food is harmful to our bodies, as evidenced in Eric Schlosser's book, *Fast Food Nation*. Our call is to be obedient, to eat the food that God created.

> *Then Jesus told his disciples, "If any man would come after me, let him deny himself and take up his cross and follow me."*
> Matthew 16:24 (RSV)

Here, Jesus was speaking in regards to dying to self. Surrender to God our will, our affections and to not seek our own happiness as the supreme object, but be willing to renounce all, and lay down our life also, if required. He is admonishing to deny our own way because He knows we want things our way. (A very popular fast-food restaurant slogan) This includes our sinful habits of indulgence in fast food, processed, and junk food. If something isn't profitable, such as junk food or overeating, and we continue in that practice, it is sin and harming our bodies.

Consider the meals of the ancients. Whatever was in their fields or growing wild, they ate. They were hunters and gatherers. They were not guided by the Food Pyramid or the media to tell them what to eat for breakfast, lunch, and dinner. For those Romans who could afford it, breakfast, eaten very early, would consist of salted bread (not the same as our bread today), milk or wine, and perhaps dried fruit, eggs or cheese. Eggs and cheese provided protein and energy. The Roman lunch was a quick meal, eaten around noon and could include salted bread or be more elaborate with fruit, salad, eggs, meat or fish, vegetable, and cheese. The Roman dinner, the main meal of the day, would be accompanied by wine, usually diluted. An ordinary upper class dinner would include meat, vegetable, egg, and fruit. Roman dessert items were figs, dates, nuts, pears, grapes, cakes, cheese, and honey. The Hebrew meals were those of the morning and evening. Jewish dietary law forbad milk and meat eaten in the same meal as revealed in Exodus 23:19. Some of the medieval and pilgrims' diet were based on the ancient Mediterranean crop triad: wheat, olives and grapes. Wine and appetizers were served. Fruits and nuts were most certainly eaten in season. Meat, such as beef, lamb and mutton, kid and goat, pork and poultry (but not turkeys, a

New World species) were mainstays along with eggs and milk.[67a]

In comparison, today's American breakfasts often consist of high sugar from doughnuts or muffins with coffee, apple, or orange juice, maybe some fried potatoes, refined grain cereal and milk. Midmorning snacks are too often bagels and cream cheese. Lunches have become quick-fix packaged and processed meals such as turkey sandwich with chips and soft drinks, "Lunchables," or fast-food meal of burgers and fries. By the afternoon the blood sugar has dropped substantially and "energy" boosting foods like candy bars are needed. A typical standard American dinner may consist of meat and potatoes, dinner roll, maybe some green beans, and topped with dessert afterwards.

In stark contrast to the foods of biblical and ancient times is the Standard American diet that consists mainly of processed foods. What is so detrimental about processed foods and how does this relate to our spiritual health?

Processed foods

Food is not what it used to be. Debbie Taylor Williams states that,

"In recent years fast foods, preservatives, additives, fried foods, and foods high in sugar, salt, and fat have taken their toll on the human body, and they cost us—physically, emotionally, and spiritually." "Lack of physical exercise and drinks substituted for water have caused the general populace to encounter health problems." "Running our gas tank on low octane fuel rather than the premium whole foods God created has caused havoc in our internal and external systems."[54]

The 1950's became the age of food processing, according to Schlosser, to "simplify the lives of American housewives" due mainly in part with the invention of refrigerators and other kitchen appliances manufactured during the late 1940's.[43] Processed food is booming business. "Seventeen thousand new products show up in the supermarket each year," adds

Pollan.[33] "The more you process any food," says Michael Pollan in *Food Rules*, "the more profitable it becomes."[34] This is especially true for the health-care industry which makes more money treating chronic diseases than preventing them.[34]

Processed food actually began during the Industrial era of the early 1900's. Hershey's chocolate, Pepsi, Kellogg's Corn Flakes, Crisco, Oreo cookies, and Wonder bread are all inventions in the early twentieth century. The refined grains became popular even earlier in the late 1880's.[9] The depression era of food scarcity gave way to a plethora of new foods on the shelves of supermarkets. Ad campaigns promoted the processed foods as "up to date." Have you noticed that many processed foods carry a health claim on the package? There you go; deception.

Processed foods are essentially dead, empty foods with no, or very little, nutrient value due to the chemical processing involved. Modern society has depended on 70% of their calories consumed through these processed refined foods compared to hunter/gatherer societies of old who consumed 26-35% of their calories from plant foods. This means they depended on animals and fats for their caloric needs.[9]

Processed foods are foods that once were living but fell into human hands and have been altered in every imaginable way, stripped of all vitamins, minerals, fiber, enzymes, phytonutrients, and antioxidants, and have added flavorings, sweeteners, and preservatives to make them last as long as possible at room temperature. Fast Food restaurants are at the top of the list of "fake" food and are the example of how far we have strayed from the real food that our ancestors ate. According to Schlosser, from the bacon, pancakes, cinnamon rolls, hamburgers, sausage, biscuits, eggs, to the fries, all the food is frozen and prepared at a factory where the foods are manufactured. Foods are assembled at the restaurants— not prepared from scratch. For instance, Taco Bell's guacamole is made at a factory in Mexico, then frozen and shipped into the United States. The beans are dehydrated and look like corn flakes.[43] Water is all that is needed to bring the foods to life.

When the natural food value of a whole food substance has been altered they are no longer whole foods. They are foods that are typically loaded with sugars and other addictive substances such as beef and other flavorings.[42] The added substances, like sugars, fool the brain into believing that it is hungry; this, in turn, drives a person to consume more calories and conserve energy. The result is a worsening cycle of sugar consumption that floods the body system with insulin and ravages the body with inflammation.[38] The other problem is that these highly processed caloric dense, "anti-nutrient" foods, actually displace the nutrients found in whole plant and animal foods.[9] The result is a body depleted of vital vitamins, minerals, essential fats, and phytonutrients.

What are some typical indications that a person is deficient in these nutrients? According to Pottenger's studies, he found symptoms such as thin, splitting, peeling nails, thin skin, or thick skin, dry brittle hair, irritability, or exhaustion were all due to essential nutrient deficiencies. He also found that poor bone and ligament development also were indicated in nutrient deficiencies.[36]

Where are these processed foods? In the aisles on shelves of grocery and convenience stores, those edible products that are boxed, canned, in a jar, or bagged have been enhanced artificially or with flavors, fat, sugar, or salt.[42] Canned foods are a relatively new invention. They did not exist in biblical times, rather were originally developed as an emergency stopgap to stave off death by starvation. Food canning was a nineteenth century French scientist's response to Napoleon Bonaparte's order to find a way for French armies to carry food. When enemy armies burned fields and food as they retreated, the French soldiers faced death by starvation. Canned foods helped them eat when no "live" food could be found.[20] Canned foods can keep a person from death, but not sustain them for a length of time.

By the end of the 1940's, fast food restaurants were just becoming popular. Well known franchises began in southern California such as Carl's Drive-In Barbeque, and In-N-Out Burger.[43] Touted for the "working-class" families, these restaurants were mainly self-service and affordable for families. In-N-Out Burger has been recognized as the highest in food quality standards............in the beginning. Even though they are known to have fresh beef, potatoes, and real milkshakes,[43] they never revealed their ingredients until Food Babe in February 2016 was able to uncover the truth. Some of what was uncovered was the following:

- GMO meat from factory farms in central California
- GMO cottonseed oil for frying the potatoes
- Hydrogenated soybean oil used in the buns
- Special "Thousand Island" type sauce made with High Fructose Corn Syrup
- Yellow dye #5
- Artificial flavors in shakes

Now approximately ten thousand new processed food products are introduced every year in the United States. Almost all of them require flavor and other additives.[43]

My father's first summer job in 1941 was working at a soda fountain in the Rexall Drug Store in Lincoln, Kansas serving malts and milkshakes. These milkshakes were made from three ingredients: whole milk ice-cream, raw milk, and strawberry syrup. As a child I can remember looking forward to Sunday evenings with my father making us his famous milkshakes. Similar to the Rexall Drug Store soda fountain, my father's homemade milkshakes consisted of three ingredients: farm fresh strawberries rather than the syrup, whole milk, and real whole milk ice cream. In stark contrast from sixty years ago, ordering a strawberry milkshake today from a popular fast food restaurant, the patron will get a drink loaded with over forty-nine chemical ingredients.[43]

The leading fast food chains have changed not just what Americans and other nations eat, but also how their food is made. The man-made fats that are added involve taking various oils and heating them to dangerously high temperatures so that the nutrients die and become something completely different and toxic to our bodies. This partially hydrogenated oil is a common ingredient in the American diet and is present in most processed and baked foods. Most of fast food is delivered to the restaurant already frozen, canned, dehydrated, or freeze-dried and completely reformulated from their original creation. Much of the taste and aroma is manufactured in chemical plants.[43] McDonald's now touts heart-healthy no trans-fats. People are eating more French fries thinking that since it isn't trans-fat, then it is okay, ignorant to the fact that anytime an oil is heated up on high heat, the oil will turn to a trans-fat.[38] The oil itself may not contain trans-fat, it is the high heat that changes it. Also, French fries are coated with sugar and beef flavoring and the food industry knows this is what makes them so addicting.[38] More people will be fooled into thinking the French fries are healthy, with little realization of the danger they are placing on their health. Deception again!

Why are processed foods so harmful? Again, they are dead foods and altered from their original state. If we eat processed foods, we are likely eating fat on fat on sugar on fat with some flavor.[42] This is not real food. The body sees these substances as foreign invaders and places a strain on the liver and immune system. Any time we have foreign invaders, the body attacks that foreign invader. This sets up a cascade of inflammation, obesity, and alters our brain chemistry. Some of the adverse effects of a continued consumption of processed fast food are: altered blood glucose, imbalance in essential fatty acid metabolism, macronutrient imbalance between carbohydrates to protein and fat, mineral deficiencies, acid/base imbalance, electrolyte imbalance, and fiber depletion.[9] A healthy functioning body should not have to depend on fiber supplements!

Studies are showing that children's academics along with nutritional status are not improving in spite of all the school improvement programs. (*Journal of Academy of Nutrition and Dietetics*) Yet the incidence of misbehavior, in the school or home setting, and the incidence of diabetes and obesity are escalating yearly. Good behavior shows that a child has learned to control his/her impulses and are not controlled by them. Scholastic excellence is a measure of a child's ability to remain mentally alert for hours. Physical fitness indicates a properly developed cardiovascular system, good eye-hand coordination, and quick reflexes. Food can enhance all of these qualities in a child and yet is rarely, if ever, taken into account in academic SST's and IEP's when the child's academics are failing and behavior is not controlled. Pottenger, in his studies, demonstrated that it is perfectly possible for a child to improve his physical fitness, health, well-being, and academic and social life after being placed on an optimal nutritional program.[36]

Parents have an additional responsibility to "Train a child up in the way they should go" as stated from Proverbs 22:6. Even as an infant or young toddler, feeding a child what they want and what tastes good such as with sugary fruits, juices, cookies, candy, cakes and pies, and highly refined carbohydrates, chips, and soda, and French fries, sets them up for the sugar addiction and junk food cycle as they age. If they learn and are trained to eat the right foods, the right amount, the right timing for eating, and what is good for them in the beginning stages of life, then this sets up a healthy pattern for the rest of their lives.

According to Mike Adams of Natural News, "The whole point of the processed food industry and the chemical products industry is to trick you into poisoning yourself," violating your own temple and seducing you into Satan's agenda of self destruction.

Food is not what it used to be. There were no fast food restaurants or packaged processed foods in biblical times. God made our food. The food eaten from the beginning of time up to the twentieth century was whole, living, or once living, foods. He made it delicious without additives or flavorings. As celebrity chef Alton Brown says, "To me, the most honor I can do to what He created is to not mar or in any way malign the creation." He continues, "No one will cook as well for you as someone who loves and cares for you." Great advice for us and an admonition to cook at home and eat home prepared food, just like people did for thousands of years before us.

Sweeteners

White Refined Sugar

Table sugar is the bleached, nutritionally-deficient byproduct of cane processing. During sugar cane processing, nearly all the minerals and vitamins end up in the blackstrap molasses that's usually fed to farm animals. (Blackstrap molasses is actually the "good" part of sugar cane juice.) Molasses is often fed to farm animals because every rancher knows that farm animals need good nutrition to stay alive. According to Dr. Rodier, sugar promotes diabetes, obesity, mood disorders and nutritional deficiencies.[38] It is also very addictive, and can cause energy receptors in the body to be desensitized so that we lose energy and need sugar to pick us up from the lethargy created by the sugar. Sugars also leaches the body of essential vitamins and upsets the balance of minerals contributing to deficiencies; especially that of magnesium and calcium.

White refined sugar is unnatural and refined from sugar cane or sugar beets. The process removes over sixty-four nutrients leaving only glucose. It is referred by many as a drug that is made from plant sources. White sugar depletes chromium, zinc, magnesium and manganese. The more sweet foods that we eat, the less room we will have for the mineral dense foods like vegetables and nuts.

In 1997 Americans devoured 7.3 billion pounds of candy, spending 23.1 billion dollars. That's equivalent to 27.3 pounds/year or six regular sized chocolate bars per week per person.[38]

In 1915, the national average intake of sugar was 15-20-pounds of sugar per person. Today, it is about 175 pounds.[38]

Sugar, the Fall Out

First, when blood sugar fluctuates from excess sugar consumption, calcium and phosphorus ratios in the blood fluctuate along with it. This increases blood calcium because calcium is being pulled from the joints and teeth in order to neutralize the toxic effects of the sugar. The longer a person's high blood sugar is out of control, the longer and more significantly the calcium and phosphorus ratios are altered. The fallout here is tooth decay and other bone and joint problems and altered parathyroid hormone. An October 2015 blog from alzheimers. net posted a link between Alzheimer's and diabetes type 2. Because diabetics produce extra insulin, the insulin gets into the brain, disrupting brain chemistry and leaves toxic proteins that poison the brain cells. The protein that forms in Alzheimer's patients is the same protein in diabetes.

Harvard trained dentist/nutritional researcher, Dr. Weston Price, D.D.S., the "Albert Einstein of Nutrition," traveled the world for six years in the 1930's studying isolated groups in Switzerland, Alaskan/ Canadian Induit, the Gaelics of the Outer Hebrides-UK, Polynesian Islanders, African tribes, New Zealand Maori, Australian Aborigines and South American Indians.[32] He determined that the diets of these primitive groups provided at least four times the water soluble vitamins, calcium, and other minerals and at least ten times the fat-soluble vitamins such as A, E, and D found in the typical Western diet of that time. Much of these nutrients were derived from diets that included butter, fatty fish, wild game and organ meats.[29] The dental health of these people was remarkable, yet they did not have dental care. Members of these groups that had "urbanized," developed much higher incidences of dental diseases, crooked teeth, joint diseases, social and emotional disorders and many other degenerative and crippling diseases.[29]

Second, refined sugar residues accumulate in the brain and nervous system and leads to carbonic poisoning and brain cell death. In January 2013, a study showed for the first time that fructose can trigger brain changes that may lead to overeating. Sugar thickens blood, has a sticky viscosity inhibiting flow into minute capillaries that supply our gums and teeth leading to dental caries. High sugar intake has also been linked with hypoglycemia, diabetes, gallstones, thyroid, menstrual, mental, emotional and behavioral disorders.

Bacteria feed off of sugars and yeast, so if we suffer from frequent bacterial infections and experience gas, irritable bowels, heartburn, bad breath, itchy skin, coated tongue, or urinary tract infections, we may possibly have an overgrowth of bacteria called, Candida Albicans. The more sugar a person consumes the happier the Candida are because they are being fed their favorite food. The best way to rid the body of this insidious problem is to starve them of their diet of sugars.

In addition to tooth decay, dental caries (cavities), and other physical disorders, another fall-out to high sugar intake is sugar addictions.

What is a sugar addiction? Addictions, according to Dr. DesMaison, are the habitual, physiological and psychological dependence on a substance or practice beyond one's voluntary control. It is the lack of ability to walk away from sweets. A person goes through withdrawals or mood swings without sugar. The thought of, "I can't live without sugar!" Or, "I just have a sweet tooth."

Refined sugars, as well as processed foods and overcooked proteins, make our cell membranes stiff and unresponsive to messages of cell communication.[38] Cells communicate in order to process and consume energy and to detoxify. If there is a miscommunication for a long period of time, then tissues, organs, and organ systems begin to malfunction.

We have a thermostat in the Hypothalamus of the brain to control our appetite, according to our metabolic needs, and diets. "The thermostat is disrupted in people with metabolic problems and cellular miscommunication," says Dr. Rodier. This is why most people find it extremely hard to lose weight or get off sugar and maintain such losses. Consuming sugars and high fructose corn syrup causes our thermostats to be set at a point where only increasing amounts of these empty foods will satiate us. This is the same mechanism by which people become addicted to drugs or alcohol. Remember, alcohol is nothing but fermented sugar. "Eating the right foods will fix your thermostat," suggests Hugo Rodier, M.D.[38]

What factors contribute to sugar addictions? First, hidden sugars are laced in everything from peanut butter, ketchup, chips, vitamins, and bread. Unless a person is an ingredient sleuth, the ingredients may be very deceptive. Instead of developing the natural taste for the product, the body develops a liking to the sweetened taste. This can lead to continued cravings for sweets and less consumption of whole foods and vegetables. According to the Journal of Nutrition in 2000, a lack of vegetables in the diet can cause our taste buds to under function and lead to zinc deficiency. Zinc deficiency causes our taste buds to only taste sweet. The sweet craving exacerbates.

A second factor begins in infancy when babies are being fed formula instead of breast milk. These formulas typically have added sugars. In addition, parents unknowingly begin prompting overeating habits by cuing the infant to finish their bottle. Babies instinctively know when to stop eating from mother's milk. When bottle feeding, it usually is the mother who decides when their baby is finished and prompts the baby to finish drinking the formula regardless of whether the baby has had his or her fill. Throwing up is a sign that the baby drank too much.

Another factor contributing to sugar addictions are parental cues. If children see parents eating and drinking sugary foods, then the child will naturally want what their parents have. Children generally will not eat better than the adults around them. Desserts used as rewards for accomplishments also sets the stage for the child to believe they are not loved unless they get a reward and then grow to expect the sugary reward instead of learning to accept praise as a satisfying reward in and of itself. Using sweets as rewards also sets the stage for children to reward themselves as adults with sweets. Restricting foods excessively is also counterproductive and can lead to binge eating. Teach children that sweets are not an everyday occurrence so that they learn to appreciate that sweets are okay once in a while or for special occasions only.

Artificial Sweeteners

First of all, "sugar-free" is not sweet free. Second, all artificial sweeteners are potent chemical agents that fool the brain cells by masking as sugar. (There you go-deception again). Sweetness normally translates to energy into the body. The sweeteners, through the taste buds, program the brain to behave as if ample sugar for its consumption has reached the body and will imminently reach it through the circulation. Since there is strict control of the level of sugar in the blood, the brain calculates the outcome of the sweetness and instructs and programs the liver not to manufacture sugar from other raw materials, but to begin storing sugar. When the sugar that was promised through the taste buds is nowhere to be found, the brain and the liver prompt a hunger sensation to find food and make good on the promise of energy. The result is a state of anxiety about food. It has been shown that people who consume artificial sweeteners ("Sugar-free" alternatives) seek food, and eat more than normal. This is part of the reason why more than 37 percent of the population are obese and why they cannot lose weight.[2] There are now some forty types of sugar used in processed food.[34] Below are a few of them:

Aspartame (Equal)

A combination of the amino acid phenylalanine, aspartic acid and methanol (wood alcohol) which are contained in Aspartame, are known to be toxic. It is found in more than 3,000 foods. Phenylalanine has been linked with carbohydrate cravings, PMS, insomnia, convulsive disorders, and mood swings by blocking production of serotonin, a neurotransmitter. So, those who drink diet coke or chew gum, most likely are serotonin depleted! It has been shown to rob the body of chromium causing severe hyperthyroid symptoms-Grave's disease, and cause irritable bowel disease and cancer. Eighty to eighty-five percent of all food related complaints to the FDA can be traced to artificial sugars.[38]

As it degrades, it forms formaldehyde—a highly toxic chemical! It is a neurotoxin and endocrine disrupter and can lead to depression and panic disorders.[38]

High Fructose Corn Syrup (HFCS)

In spite of the deceptive commercials that tout, "sugar is sugar," this is not the same fructose that is in fruit. HFCS contains the synthetic form of fructose and is toxic to the body. This sugar is in many commercial processed foods, cocktail drinks, sweetened drinks, soft drinks, in children's vitamins, and food bars even under the disguise of FOS or inulin or corn sugar. HFCS is a highly processed liquid sugar extracted with the chemical solvent glutaraldehyde and frequently contaminated with mercury. It is also linked to diabetes, obesity, and mood disorders. HFCS is used in sodas and countless grocery items, including things you wouldn't suspect like pizza sauce and salad dressings. According to Ramiel Nagel, the prevalence of the dangerous high fructose corn syrup in our foods is due to government subsidies to the corn industry that makes fructose cheaper to produce than natural sugar.[29] Again, deception and food politics!

Saccharin (Sweet N Low)

Saccharin is the oldest of artificial sweeteners and was discovered in 1879 at Johns Hopkins University. This is a synthetic compound derived from coal tar. It is three hundred times sweeter than sugar, and was placed on the FDA list of carcinogens since 1977, but removed in 2000. Saccharin is reported to have little effect on blood sugar, unlike sugar.

Sucralose (Splenda)

This is an altered sugar molecule-a Chloride radical added to a sugar (sucrose) molecule similar to table salt NaCl. It is six hundred times sweeter than sugar and associated with shrunken thymus glands, enlarged liver and kidneys, atrophy of lymph follicles in the spleen and thymus, increased small intestine weight, reduced growth rate, decreased RBC counts, hyperplasia of the pelvis, extended pregnancy, spontaneous abortion, decreased fetal body weights and placental weights, and diarrhea. But, it is reported to have little or no effect on blood sugar!

Remember all sweets have an effect on blood sugar. Especially avoid white sugar, jelly, candy bars, palm sugar, fructose, HFCS, brown rice syrup, maltodextrin, maltose, sucrose, dextrose, sucralose, caramel coloring, corn sweetener, hexitol, aspartame, and saccharine. And, if a person craves sweets, it could be an indication of a sugar addiction. As expressed by Charles Stanley, "Those who can't say no to their own desires end up enslaved to them."[46] All sweeteners should be used in moderation.

Alternatives to Artificial Sweeteners

Honey

My child, eat honey because it is good. Honey from the honeycomb tasted sweet.

Proverbs 24:13

If you find honey don't eat too much. Too much of it will make you sick.

Proverbs 25:16

Honey was prevalent in ancient times. According to Loren Cordain, sugar was introduced about 6,000 years ago in India. It didn't become available to the masses until around 1798 A.D.[9] In biblical times people ate sweets. We find scriptures that reveal sweets; mostly regarding honey and dates. Nevertheless, the sweet pastries prepared then and even as recently as a hundred years ago, used whole unrefined grain and honey, compared to today's refined grain flour and processed sugar.

God created flowering plants to produce nectar which contains a combination of sucrose and glucose in different ratios. The bees that He created gather the nectar from the flowers and store it in their special collecting chambers. The enzymes in these chambers degrade or split the sucrose into fructose and glucose; a perfect ratio required for the formation of liver glycogen and allows it to pass into the bloodstream within minutes. Glycogen is the primary fuel for the brain.

Raw honey has healing qualities and has been used for centuries to heal wounds and insect bites, prevent scarring, treat infections, improve immune system functioning, stabilize blood sugar levels, and provide quick energy. It also has antimicrobial properties.

Unlike sugar, it has only 25 calories per teaspoon. Raw unfiltered honey is nutrient rich because it has not been processed with pasteurization and contains Vitamins A, B -Complex, C, D, E, Beta-carotene and K, Magnesium, Sulfur, Phosphorus, Iron, Calcium, Potassium, Iodine, Sodium, Copper and Magnesium. Additionally honey contains a rich supply of live enzymes. Three to five tablespoons taken in divided doses a day is recommended for optimum health benefits. Below are a few other scripture references to authenticate honey's important uses:

And I am come down to deliver them out of the hand of the Egyptians, and to bring them up out of that land unto a good land, unto a land flowing with milk and honey; unto the place of the Canaanites, and the Hittites, and the Amorites, and the Perizzites, and the Hivites, and the Jebusites.

Exodus 3:8

A land of wheat, and barley, and vines, and fig trees, and pomegranates; a land of oil olive, and honey;

Deuteronomy 8:8

My son, eat honey, because [it is] good; and the honeycomb, [which is] sweet to your taste:

Proverbs 24:13

And the same John had his raiment of camel's hair, and a leathern girdle about his loins; and his meat was locusts and wild honey.

Matthew 3:4

Honey isn't what it used to be. According to Andrew Schneider of Food Safety News, three-fourths of honey sold in the United States isn't what bees produce. The pollen has been filtered out. This ultra filtering is a procedure where honey is heated, watered down, and forced at high pressure to remove the pollen. Without the pollen there is no tracking of the honey's origin, and no beneficial nutrients. In fact, most of the honey that comes from China has been found to contain animal antibiotics. The quality of the honey through ultra filtration is diminished and is "a deceptive and unethical practice," reports Schneider. The majority of honey sold in frequented grocery stores, grocery outlets and clubs now contain this ultra filtered processed honey. Sixty percent of ultra filtered honey used in baked goods, beverages, sauces, and processed foods comes from foreign honey sold to the food industry. Unless you are purchasing from a beekeeper, Farmer's Market, or food Co-op, "you are at risk for adulterated honey," remarks Schneider.

Agave Nectar

This is a high-fructose-containing food, similar looking to an aloe plant, disguised as a healthy food. It contains equal or more of fructose corn syrup. Research has shown that it is not a raw or unrefined product as marketed. This is not necessarily a health food. According to Theresa Dale, PhD in one of her posts, "The process in which the agave starch is converted into refined fructose and then sold as the sweetener agave nectar is through an enzymatic and chemical conversion that refines, clarifies, heats, chemically alters, centrifuges, and filters the non-sweet starch into a highly refined sweetener, fructose." "In my testing of various brands of agave, I have found that NONE of them are suitable for a healthy diet." In contrast, according to K.C. Craichy, in moderation, organic agave can be part of a healthy diet if used in combination with food including healthy proteins, fats, fiber and when balanced with other natural sugars in the diet. Agave nectar is not a good option for use in beverages.

Barley Malt Syrup

This is a whole grain sweetener made from sprouted or hot air-dried barley. It is high in complex carbohydrates leaving little impact on blood sugar.

Erythritol

Erythritol is a sweetener made from sugar alcohols and is used in different foods as an artificial sweetener. It is also formulated in labs using yeast fermentation. According to the FDA, it is safe for consumption by diabetic patients because it does not raise insulin levels. Some bulk foods like diet sodas and sugar-free cereals, cakes and juices are sweetened with erythritol.[57]

Erythritol is not as sweet as sugar, requiring that more be used to sweeten foods and this is what can lead to overuse. Even when it is used in foods, minimal erythritol health risks are present—only such benefits as longer freshness, softer dough and even the control of crystallization. Some health effects are digestive complications such as bloating and gas; common in most sugar alcohols.[57]

In 1999, erythritol was reviewed by the WHO/FAO Joint Expert Committee on Food Additives and was given the highest food safety grading possible. On the other hand, a study by Louisiana Tech University in 2011 showed that erythritol combined with fructose increased carbohydrate malabsorption.[64]

Maltitol

This is a sugar substitute known as a sugar alcohol. Sugar alcohols, although do not pose an impact on blood sugar like regular sugars do with diabetics, but have their own inherent risk. The chemical structure is similar to that of alcohol and sugar. Even though a person cannot become inebriated or have an insulin surge after consumption, the intestines can be affected with gas, bloating, or diarrhea due to the fermenting of the sugar alcohol. This substance is one of the substitutes some companies use as a replacement for high fructose corn syrup and is commonly added to children's vitamins.[17] Use in moderation.

Maple Syrup

Maple syrup is sold by Grade. Grade B organic maple syrup is the best because it has retained many of the beneficial nutrients. These are organic acids, amino acids, minerals, vitamin A and B vitamins. Many generic maple syrups may contain formaldehyde residue even though the practice of using formaldehyde pellets to keep tap holes in trees open is currently forbidden. Use organic Grade B only.

Molasses

This is a byproduct of beet or cane sugar. It has many valuable nutrients like iron and potassium and is easily recognized by the body.

Sorghum

A concentrated juice of the millet-like sorghum plant, it has a lighter and fruitier flavor than molasses. It has high protein and mineral content.

Stevia

Stevia comes from the small shrub found in Brazil and Paraguay. Native Guarini tribes used the leaves as a sweetener for many centuries. It is one hundred to three hundred times sweeter than sugar, but does not have an effect on blood sugar metabolism. Some studies have even shown a decrease in glucose levels among adults with normal blood sugars levels when Stevia has been ingested.

It is touted as the "safe" sweetener, but should still be used with caution. Some brands extract components of the stevia leaf and these are dangerous and overly processed and likely cause imbalances to the glandular system. Do not use stevia that is stored in glycerin or combined with sucralose. The glycerin could be made from a petrochemical and sucralose, as stated above, is nothing more than Splenda.

Sucanat

This is an unrefined dehydrated or evaporated sugar cane juice with a molasses flavor. It is high in simple sugars, yet retains the sugar cane's nutrients._

Xylitol

Xylitol is a sugar alcohol and not simply a sugar. It is metabolized in the liver. According to author Ramiel Nagel, the Journal of the American Dental Association claims Xylitol stops cavities. These anti-cavity properties are purported to depend on the fact that bacteria cannot digest sugar alcohols and convert them into acids. However, bacteria and acids are not the primary culprits in tooth decay. Diet is!

Other sweeteners are sorbitol and mannitol. These and the other sugar alcohols are usually well tolerated by the vast majority of people and have health promoting properties including prebiotic and low glycemic impact, but as with all sugars, use in moderation.

Salt

What about salt? Was it used in Biblical times and how does it compare with today's salt?

> *And every offering of your grain offering you shall season with salt; you shall not allow the salt of the covenant of your God to be lacking from your grain offering. With all your offerings you shall offer salt.*
>
> Leviticus 2:13

> *......but the water is bad and the ground barren." And he said, "Bring me a new bowl, and put salt in it. So they brought [it] to him. Then he went out to the source of the water, and cast in the salt there, and said, "Thus says the Lord: I have healed this water; from it there shall be no more death or barrenness."*
>
> 2 Kings 2:19-21

> *Can that which is unsavory be eaten without salt? Or is there [any] taste in the white of an egg?*
>
> Job 6:6

> *Salt [is] good: but if the salt has lost its flavor, how shall it be seasoned?*
>
> Luke 14:34

Salt is put in all processed food to preserve it and has the ability to preserve food. It was a critical element in the growth and development of early civilization as referenced in the scriptural passages above. It eliminated the dependence on the seasonal availability of food and it allowed travel over long distances.

Salt contains sodium, an electrolyte which is crucial to water balance in the body. Sodium is the major positive ion (cation) in fluid outside of cells. The chemical notation for sodium is Na+. When combined with chloride, the resulting substance is table salt. Excess sodium (such as that obtained from dietary sources) is excreted in the urine. Sodium regulates the total amount of water in the body and the transmission of sodium into and out of individual cells also plays a role in critical body functions. Many processes in the body, especially in the brain, nervous system, and muscles, require electrical signals for communication. The movement of sodium is critical in generation of these electrical signals. Too much or too little sodium, therefore, can cause cells to malfunction, and extremes in the blood sodium levels (too much or too little) can be fatal.[62]

Not only was salt valuable to keep the body's electrolytes in balance but was also used to control infections. Even during the civil war, salt poultices were placed on wounds to prevent infection. However, salt was difficult to obtain unless a person lived near a coast, and so it was a highly valued trade item. Salt was taken from the sea and filtered through large apothecaries and placed in the sun to remove the impurities. It is commonly believed that Roman soldiers were at certain times paid with salt. In the Old Testament, Mosaic Law called for salt to be added to all burnt animal sacrifices (Leviticus 2:13). The Book of Ezra (550 BC to 450 BC) associated accepting salt from a person with being in that person's service.[67]

You are the salt of the earth.

Matthew 5:13

Jesus said this in order to show his disciples how valuable they were, and this saying is commonly used today to describe someone who is of particular value to society. In addition, the preservative quality of salt is in view here to show how the disciples were called to preserve the society and the world around them from moral decay.

During more modern times, it became more profitable to sell salted food than to sell pure table salt.[67] Iodized salt is table salt mixed with a minute amount of various iodine-containing salts. The ingestion of iodide prevents iodine deficiency. Worldwide, iodine deficiency affects about two billion people and is the leading preventable cause of mental retardation. Iodine deficiency also causes thyroid gland problems, including endemic goiter. In many countries, iodine deficiency is a major public health problem that can be cheaply addressed by iodization of salt.[69]

Iodine is a micronutrient that is naturally present in the food supply in many regions. However, where natural levels of iodine in the soil are low and the iodine is not taken up by vegetables, iodine is added to salt to provide the small but essential amount needed by humans. However, iodide-treated table salt slowly loses its iodine content through the process of oxidation and evaporation.[69]

In the U.S. in the early 20th century, goiters (caused by iodine deficiency) were especially prevalent in the region around the Great Lakes and the Pacific Northwest. David Murray Cowie, a professor of pediatrics at the University of Michigan, led the U.S. to adopt the Swiss practice of adding sodium iodide or potassium iodide to table and cooking salt. On May 1, 1924, iodized salt was sold commercially in Michigan. By the fall of 1924, Morton Salt Company began distributing iodized salt nationally.[69]

In areas where there is little iodine in the diet, typically remote inland areas and semi-arid equatorial climates where no marine foods are eaten, iodine deficiency gives rise to hypothyroidism (symptoms of which are extreme fatigue), goiter, mental slowing, depression, weight gain, and low basal body temperatures. Iodine deficiency is the leading cause of preventable mental retardation, a result that occurs primarily when babies or small children are rendered hypothyroidic by a lack of the element iodide. The addition of iodine to table salt has largely eliminated this problem in the wealthier nations, but, as of March 2006, iodine deficiency remained a serious public health problem in the developing world.

Table salt often has iodide as well as anticaking ingredients. Typically anticaking agents are not soluble in water and form an unwanted precipitate. Our bodies react to these foreign substances with inflammation. For years doctors have told patients to cut back or cut out salt due to hardening of the arteries or for blood pressure control. It is not the salt which creates disease, but rather the dirt and excipients in the salt. National policies that advise restricting sodium (salt) intake to reduce the risk of hypertension might not provide the anticipated cardiovascular benefits and may even be detrimental to health.[10] It might be necessary to include iodine, under the supervision of a doctor or health care practitioner, as a supplement if salt consumption has been limited or if one is using salt without iodine.

Though salt intake was high in ancient civilizations, high blood pressure was not recorded as a disease in biblical times. In comparison, the salt today is mined from the ground and not filtered as the ancients did. However, eliminating salt disrupts the electrolyte balance. It is the balance of salt in the fluid of our body that creates a pressure differential which moves nutrients through cell membranes. This osmotic pressure differential is like having billions of little pumps moving important nutrients throughout our body.[10] It is the processed foods that need to be eliminated; not salt indiscriminately.

Salt today is still utilized as a preservative and flavoring. Now we have Himalayan, Kosher, black salt, sea salt, and Celtic Sea Salt that are beneficial options as long as they are sand free and without anticaking ingredients. Natural sources of iodine include sea life, such as kelp and certain seafood, as well as plants grown on iodine-rich soil.

With the added sodium, artificial sweeteners, processed foods, and toxic stressors so prevalent, is it any wonder we have gotten out of balance?

5

......

God's Immune System Design Gone Awry

By God's design, we have a healthy, normally functioning immune system with checks and balances that keep us from developing allergies, asthma, rheumatoid, chronic fatigue, cancer, and the like. In simplistic terms we have been given Natural Killer Cells. The two types of lymphocytes that are killer cells are the cytotoxic T Helper cells (Th1) produced in the thymus gland. These cells control the initiation or suppression of the body's immune reactions and regulate other immune cells. Th1 cells promote specialized cell-mediated (inside the cell) immunity and are the special forces that defend the body. They produce only as many germ-zapping antibodies as necessary to stop an invader. The other is Th2, which produces a mass response to infection in the form of proteins called antibodies that are secreted into body fluids by B-lymphocytes.[39] The Th2 cells are the army and navy defenders in the body. Both types contain granules filled with potent chemicals, and both types kill invading antigens on contact. The killer binds to its target, aims its weapons, and delivers a burst of lethal chemicals. The main difference is that Th1 forces attacks abnormal cells and microorganisms at the site of infection, inside the cells, and Th2 cells trigger the mass production of antibodies to neutralize foreign invaders and substances outside of cells.[39]

It is not a matter of killing off all bacteria to keep healthy We need bacteria. God created us with good and bad bacteria and when we acquire too many microbials, the good bacteria are designed to take over in the healing process; not eradicate all bacteria. In a healthy person, this is the natural process our immune system accomplishes to keep us healthy. It is when our immune system is compromised that this process is hampered. In 2006, the Journal of Clinical Gastroenterology disclosed that eating foods high in refined sugars, or chemical additives, alters the delicate balance of friendly intestinal flora, which is the basis of the immune system in the intestines.

We were created with an incredible organ called the liver which functions as a filtering system for toxins and other waste. Toxins enter our bodies through the skin, lungs, mouth, or gastrointestinal tract. The antigens, the toxins, the uninvited guests, eventually have to confront the liver where they are dispatched in one of three ways: locked away into the liver itself, sent on for elimination to the kidneys, or stored away in fat cells. If our bodies are weak or the elimination channels of the kidneys or respiratory system are blocked and these toxins are not excreted in a timely manner, they build up.

Dr. Samuel Epstein in 1944 predicted that one-third of us will get cancer in our lifetimes as a result of exposures to synthetic chemicals which would tax and overwork the liver. Prior to the 1940's, synthetic chemicals never existed.[12] Our bodies were not designed to protect themselves against an overabundance of chemical onslaughts which can tax our liver's detoxification process. Because of this, our body systems begin to fail to process and remove most of these accumulated toxins once they have entered our bodies.[12]

All toxins, chemicals and other stressors, compromise the immune system. God did not design our bodies to operate at optimum levels on junk food, fast food, chemically laden, or prepackaged foods prepared in microwave ovens. He also did not design His food to contain antibiotics either. During the last century we have seen an influx of antibiotics used in livestock. Brad Spellberg, M.D. states that the use of antibiotics in livestock is the promoter of antibiotic resistant problem as the antibiotics enter human circulation through the food consumption. "Physicians that overuse antibiotics for viral rather than bacterial infections also contributes to the spread of drug resistance," Spellberg continues. God's laws that govern our entire human nature, including our health, bring consequences when violated.[39] I believe the staggering cancer statistics and drug resistance bacteria are two such consequences.

In 2007, a local newspaper reported that by 2010 cancer would overtake heart disease as the number one killer. According to the New York Times in October of 2011, heart disease is no longer the leading killer of Americans under age 85. Cancer is.

In fact, as Jane Brody reported, cancer deaths surpassed heart disease in people under 85 as far back as 1999. But until the American Cancer Society compiled its annual statistical report for this year, no one had looked before at deaths among people in this very large age group, which accounts for 98.4 percent of the population.

Current research has determined that the immune system is compromised by several factors. The following are some of these factors.

1.   Poor Nutrition

Besides processed food consumption, another cause of compromised immune system and poor nutrition is from **depleted topsoil**. For thousands of years and up to one hundred years ago the topsoil was twelve inches in depth and rich in beneficial bacteria, other organisms, and vital nutrients. Today it is maybe six inches deep. How did this happen? Remember the Black Blizzards and Dust storms of the 1930s in middle America? The Dust Bowl was a period of severe dust storms causing major ecological and agricultural damage to American and Canadian prairie lands from 1930 to 1936 (in some areas until 1940). The phenomenon was caused by severe drought coupled with decades of extensive farming without crop rotation, fallow fields, cover crops, or other techniques to prevent wind erosion. Deep plowing of the virgin topsoil of the Great Plains had displaced the natural deep-rooted grasses that normally kept the soil in place and trapped moisture even during periods of drought and high winds.

But during the drought of the 1930s, without the natural anchors from the grasses to keep the soil in place, it dried, turned to dust, and blew away eastward and southward in large dark clouds. Clouds blackened the sky reaching all the way to East Coast cities of New York and Washington, D.C. Much of the soil ended up deposited in the Atlantic Ocean, carried by prevailing winds, which were in part created by the dry and bare soil conditions. These enormous dust storms were given names such as "Black Blizzards" and "Black Rollers." The storms often reduced visibility to a few feet. The Dust Bowl affected 100,000,000 acres centered on the panhandles of Texas and Oklahoma, and parts of New Mexico, Colorado, and Kansas.[67a]

The topsoil was blown away. All the minerals and nutrients that had previously built up in the topsoil vanished in these agricultural fields of the Midwest. According to Fitzgerald, an estimated 85 percent of nutrients were removed from crop soils in North America during the twentieth century.[12] Millions of acres of farmland became useless as crops would not grow in this shallow soil, and hundreds of thousands of people were forced to leave their homes; many of these families migrated to California and other states, where they found economic conditions slightly better during the Great Depression than those they had left.

In addition, after World War II the natural organisms in the soil were displaced as a result of chemical farming and pesticide usage by commercial agriculture business. For thousands of years these beneficial microorganisms were consumed as we ate the produce. Compared to today, the soil is essentially sterile and has contributed to depleted beneficial gastrointestinal bacterial, termed, "gut flora."[39]

2.   Decreased Minerals

Another cause of the compromised immune system is the **decreased mineral** content in foods because topsoil only contains three minerals-Nitrogen, Potassium, and Phosphorus. When there is deficient soil then there are deficient plants. When the plants are deficient then the food is deficient. When the food is deficient then we have deficient humans. And consequently, when the plants are deficient, they are more prone to diseases and pests. Subsequently, the pesticides have to be used to kill the pests, making the plants and foods unhealthier to eat.[6] A vicious cycle.

Take current potato production. Due to the popular demand of French fries, potatoes are grown in one crop. There is virtually no crop rotation and the crop relies heavily on chemical fertilizers, pesticides, fungicides, herbicides to grow.[43]

According to Fitzgerald, when whole wheat is refined into white flour for white bread, 95 percent fiber is lost, 84 percent iron, 95 percent vitamin E, 82 percent manganese, 80 percent niacin, and 81 percent vitamin B12 are lost.[12] Further processing from irradiating insects and microorganisms also destroys vitamins and essential nutrients in the food.[12]

3.   Week-old Food

Third, **week-old food and highly cooked foods** causes the enzymes in the food to be destroyed.[8] Enzymes are responsible for the biochemical reactions that bring food to maturity and help digest food. When the body is depleted of enzymes this leads to inflammation because the body treats destroyed enzymes as foreign and launches an attack. Digestive ailments are a major health problem. Look at the billions of dollars spent on antacids every year.

Food may travel some 250,000 miles before it gets to a grocery store. By the time it gets to us it is a week old. If it sits in the house for another week, it is two weeks old by the time we eat it. By the next day eating those leftovers how much nutritional value is still left? 40%? Possibly less. If we ate more than 51% cooked food, our body would react as if it was being invaded by a foreign organism. If our diet was 51% raw, our body would have no leukocytosis (White Blood Cell reaction). To alleviate immune reactions we need to eat more raw food such as salads and vegetables, and take pancreatic digestive enzymes when eating cooked foods.[8]

4.   Chemically Laden Foods

The fourth cause of compromised immune system comes from

chemically laden and fake foods. These foods are filled with pesticides (because plants are deficient in minerals, which brings bugs), herbicides, fungicides, preservatives, colors, flavor enhancers, environmental pollutants, additives, to name a few. In a 2013 ABC news report, food fraud was up 60 percent. Pomegranate juice was the most popular target for food fraud. Studies found pomegranate juice diluted with other juices or synthetic pomegranate. Lemon juice, coffee, olive oil, tea, and spices were also on this list of tampering using dilutions, colors, and fillers. Another example is a food based company that petitioned to have a "safe" anti-microbial preservative instead of sodium benzoate added to their foods. **BactoCEASE** extends the shelf life of the foods, but the health consequences to long term consumption has led to brain damage, personality disorders, gastrointestinal problems, autism, and migraines. Sodium benzoate alone has been known to break down the immune system.

5.   <u>Genetically Modified/Genetically Engineered foods</u>

Genetically Modified Foods (GMO) is another factor in our compromised immune system. Genetically modified organisms have had specific changes introduced into their DNA by genetic engineering techniques. Certain "favorable" traits of one organism are inserted into another organism's genes which permanently alters the second organism's DNA. The justification for this is less crop loss from pests, and more crop yields. Some crops that are genetically modified include soybean, corn, canola, rice, and cotton seed oil. Mercola, M.D., reports that cows have been genetically engineered to create something more akin to human breast milk in an effort to make cow's milk more nutritious. Genetically engineered (GE), synonymous with GMO, corn and soy have been shown to reduce fertility in animals. And GE crops are heavily sprayed with the common weed killer Roundup.[27] Not only are these foods far removed from their original design, the body does not recognize these as real food. As a consequence, the GMO food stays in the gut and ferments. Then the body launches an attack on this fake food.

In addition, GMO foods contain heavy amounts of pesticide residues which can lead to endocrine diseases such as infertility. This pesticide residue is called Glyphosphate. It has the ability to throw off the delicate hormonal balance that governs the reproductive cycle.[27] Although industries making GE/GMO foods insist the foods are safe and no different from conventionally grown varieties, the research does not support their claim.[27] Some researched health effects from GE/GMO food consumption are lung damage, cancer, altered DNA, arthritis, osteoporosis, Sudden Death Syndrome, and inflammatory bowel disease. Ninety-three percent of soybeans, 93% of canola, 93% of cottonseed oil, and 95% sugar beets are genetically engineered; remember, they all come with pesticide residue of Round up.[27] Thirty-eight percent of the corn and 80 percent of soy planted in the United States are genetically engineered and derivatives of these crops show up in 70% of all processed foods, according to Fitzgerald.[12] Our food is not what it used to be. We are being deceived —again. Fortunately, due to demands of the public new rulings are being enacted to enforce the labeling of these GMO products.

6.   Highly Refined Carbohydrates

The sixth reason for compromised immune systems in our society is due to **highly refined carbohydrates** and starches from breads, pasta, cakes, cookies, cereals, and bagels. These refined carbohydrates are devoid of bodybuilding nutritional elements. B vitamins for example, which are removed during the refining process, are needed to help breakdown carbohydrates. The empty calories deplete the body's reserves of nutrients. As long as people eat poorly every day, they will be ill in a low grade manner while not noticing any immediate effect. Dietary indiscretions precipitate the resurgence of symptoms.[19]

7.   Acidic diet

Additionally, an **excessively acid diet** stemming from such combinations as meat and potatoes, refined grains, soda and coffee, sweets and processed food consumption on a frequent basis leads to poor health and compromised immune systems. "A well-tuned body doesn't run well on inferior fuel," says M.T. Morter, M.D.

Potential hydrogen, or pH, is the measure of the relative acidity or alkalinity of a solution. Our body, by God's design, is alkaline, except in the stomach, yet acid-producing by function. Cells operate in an alkaline environment, yet acid is produced as they function. Our bodies eliminate acid through the function of various organs. Acid from food must be neutralized before it can be eliminated.

Dietary acid ash, which forms when food is burned leaving an ash residue from food after metabolizing, is eliminated through the kidneys. This residue can be measured for its mineral content. These mineral are chloride, phosphorus, or sulfur. In this process, these vital minerals are lost. Acid ash from foods can be eliminated through the kidneys and bowels, but it must first be neutralized through buffering. Otherwise, it would burn sensitive tissue on their way through the digestive tract. Pain or burning on urination, or heartburn, is an indicator that the reserves of neutralizing minerals such as calcium are exhausted and that the body has adapted the way it functions for survival, not comfort.

Alkaline-ash foods on the other hand, are foods that leave high concentrations of magnesium, calcium, and potassium in their ash. These foods are called "alkaline-ash" because these minerals are used to form alkaline compounds (called bases) in the body including magnesium hydroxide, calcium hydroxide, and potassium hydroxide.

Due to the acid producing nature of processed and sweet foods after consumption, these foods contribute to the process of sodium, potassium, calcium, magnesium and other acid-neutralizing chemicals to be used up in preventing tissue damage. These chemical elements are drawn from the tissues and must be replaced or deficiencies will occur, which can then lead to disease process and eventually kidney burnout and possibly kidney stones. The displacement of fruits and vegetables by grain based diets also shifts our body into yielding acid. If we don't replace the minerals from fruits and vegetables, our valuable reserve of alkaline minerals will vanish and our body will become acidic. When sodium reserves are used up, then the body will start to rob calcium from the bones. Osteoporosis develops when "your calcium has gone off to play hero and bail you out of the mess caused by your dietary habits," says Dr. Morter. Other diseases promoted by acidosis are diabetes and hypertension.[9]

Other reasons our system has gone awry can be attributed to infection, inflammation, toxicity, oxidation with uncontrolled free-radicals roaming about, trauma from accidents, X-ray radiation poisoning from airport scanners, mammograms, dental or other X-rays, or nuclear fallout, accidents, and stress -either emotional, physical, or mental.

With all the above toxic exposures, food adulteration, and diet choices, is it any wonder how we have become dis-ordered and have compromised immune systems? According to Ann Wigmore, the food you eat can either be the safest and most powerful form of medicine, or the slowest form of poison. We all have choices to make and thankfully we have a God who has given us free will. We have a summons to choose that which is best for our body, our mind, and our spiritual life, so that we can faithfully live out our mission, or calling, in life.

6

. . . . . .

Improving our Health

I have attempted to uncover how and why we got out of balance; now what? There are numerous ways to improve our health. Purges, fasting, and baths were common ancient remedies and still useful today. Numerous detoxification methods are available to improve our health. Nutritional support with herbs or homeopathic remedies, saunas, Epsom Salt baths, colon irrigation, coffee enemas, skin brushing (using a loofa before showering), or ionic cleanses are a few such examples.

Detoxification is the process of pulling toxins out of tissue binding sites in the body. It is also about giving your body a break so it can do what it needs to do to stay healthy. As referenced from Randall Fitzgerald, by eliminating toxins from food and chemical toxins from the body through detoxification, the body's own regenerative chemistry is magnified and the immune system is strengthened.[12]

With today's onslaught of toxicity, it is critical to undergo some form of detoxification program at least once a year. An effective detoxification program is garnered through certified nutritionists or healthcare practitioners who will guide participants through the program. One sustainable program that I recommend is centered on sound science-based nutrition and takes into account those with food sensitivities and factors in homeopathic drainage remedies. Any kind of cleanse or detox program may produce detox symptoms. These are the result of the body mobilizing toxins and circulating them through the body. Symptoms could include headaches, dizziness, emotional shifts, flare up of previous complaints, rashes, or others, which is why any special detoxification program should be carried out with supervision from a licensed health care practitioner.

Skin brushing involves using a loofa in the shower. This process removes dead skin cells and stimulates circulation.

Epsom salt baths involve soaking in a tub for twenty minutes. (Add Peppermint Oil to the salts to intensify the detox effect.) Twenty minutes in a bath with Essential Oils and Epsom Salts equals one quart of toxins eliminated due to osmotic properties drawing toxins out. Drinking water afterwards further enhances this process.

Coffee enemas- Enemas date back to Egyptian practices in 1500 B.C. They were known to employ this practice monthly because they believed that disease was "engendered by superfluities of the food;" wisdom from the ancients still applicable for today! Coffee began to be the preferred ingredient around 1920's when German scientists found that the caffeine solution could open the bile ducts and stimulate the production of bile in the liver, dilate blood vessels and counter inflammation of the gut.

Salt Flushes are very thorough colonics that cleanse the stomach, small intestines and colon and are safe when used accordingly.

Deep relaxation daily. Rest is scriptural as shown in the following sample of scriptures:

Six days you are to do your work, but on the seventh day you shall cease [from labor] in order that your ox and your donkey may rest, and the son of your female slave, as well as your stranger, may refresh themselves.

Exodus 23:12 (NAS)

Come to me, all you who labor and are heavy laden, and I will give you rest.

Matthew 11:28

Fasting

Our culture now revels in feasting, and not just at the traditional holiday occasions. It is rare that the average American experiences true hunger like that felt in the third world countries. Don Colbert, M.D. in his book, *Toxic Relief* states, "Sickness and degenerative disease are usually nature's way of telling you that your body is toxic and needs to be cleansed."[7] Because our bodies were not designed to handle all the toxic burdens and stresses we are experiencing today, fasting is a safe, natural, and powerful way to cleanse the body from the toxic waste that has accumulated. Fasting also allows the body to heal by giving it a rest from all the energy it has expended from dealing with toxins.

Biblically there is direction for fasting as we see below in these scriptural references. It is healthy for a time to fast or detoxify the body to help us grow spiritually and to regenerate the body and energize the cells.[7] There were many reasons as well as instructions God gave for fasting.

Moreover when you fast, do not be like the hypocrites, with a sad countenance. For they disfigure their faces that they may appear to men to be fasting. Assuredly, I say to you, they have their reward.

Matthew 6:16

Here we see instructions to fast in quiet; to not bring attention to ourselves.

And when he had fasted forty days and forty nights, afterward he was hungry.

Matthew 4:2

And there was one Anna, a prophetess, the daughter of Phanuel, of the tribe of Asher. She was of a great age, and had lived with a husband seven years from her virginity; and this woman was a widow of about eighty-four years, who did not depart from the temple, but served God with fastings and prayers night and day.

Luke 2:36-37

So he was there with the Lord forty days and forty nights; he neither ate bread, nor drank water. And he wrote on the tablets the words of the covenant, the Ten Commandments.

Exodus 34:28

And he was three days without sight, and neither ate nor drank.

Acts 9:9

These few passages above affirm that fasting is a Biblical principle; Jesus fasted, Anna fasted, Moses fasted, Paul fasted.

In searching scripture, fasting was done for a time and purpose. Jehoshphat's declaration in 2 Chronicles 20 is another instance of fasting for a purpose. Jehoshaphat was informed that a great multitude was coming against him. The first thing he did was to turn to God and proclaim a fast throughout Judah. His people came in support of their king through prayer. Victory prevailed because of this action.

The Bible describes several types of fasting used for physical, mental and spiritual reasons; public and private.

"Go, gather together all the Jews who are present in Shushan, and fast for me, and neither eat nor drink for three days, night or day. My maids and I will fast likewise. And so I will go to the king, which is against the law; and if I perish, I perish."

Esther 4:16

Esther participated in a three day total fast from all foods and liquids (critical fast) for deliverance and divine favor.[7] She could have given in to self-despair and turned to the comforts of food and drink, but instead chose God's directive with humility. Historically, fasting was used when facing a difficult decision, worry, or spiritual concern. It was understood as a humbling of oneself before God and directed toward God, not toward the self.

> *In those days I, Daniel, was mourning three full weeks. I ate no pleasant food, no meat or wine came into my mouth, nor did I anoint myself at all, till three whole weeks were fulfilled.*
>
> Daniel 10:2-3

Daniel used fasting as a preparation for divine inspiration and knowledge.

> *"Please test your servants for ten days, and let them give us vegetables to eat and water to drink. Then let our countenances be examined before you, and the countenances of the young men who eat the portion of the king's delicacies; and as you see fit, so deal with your servants." So he consented with them in this matter, and tested them ten days. And at the end of ten days their countenance appeared better and fatter in flesh than all the young men who ate the portion of the king's delicacies.*
>
> Daniel 1:12-15

Daniel 1:12-15 was a 10 day modified food intake abstinence diet, because the purpose was to abstain from gentile pagan food.

> *Why have we fasted, they say, and You have not seen? Why have we afflicted our souls, and You take no notice? In fact, in the day of your fast you find pleasure, and exploit all your laborers. Indeed you fast for strife and debate, and to strike with the fist of wickedness. You will not fast as you do this day, to make your voice heard on high. Is it a fast that I have chosen, a day for a man to afflict his soul? Is it to bow down his head like a bulrush, and to spread out sackcloth and ashes? Would you call this a fast,*

and an acceptable day to the Lord? Is this not the fast that I have chosen: To loose the bonds of wickedness, to undo the heavy burdens, to let the oppressed go free, and that you break every yoke? Is it not to share your bread with the hungry, and that you bring to your house the poor who are cast out; When you see the naked, that you cover him, and not hide yourself from your own flesh? Then your light shall break forth like the morning, your healing shall spring forth speedily, and your righteousness shall go before you; The glory of the Lord shall be your rear guard. Then you shall call, and the Lord will answer; You shall cry, and He will say, "Here I am."

Isaiah 58:3-9

Isaiah shows us we need to have the proper motive whenever we embark on a fasting.

Then I proclaimed a fast there, at the river of Ahava, that we might humble ourselves before our God, to seek from him the right way for us, and for our little ones, and all our possessions.

Ezra 8:21

Then as he lay and slept under a broom (juniper) tree, suddenly an angel touched him, and said unto him, "Arise and eat." Then he looked, and there by his head was a cake baked on coals, and a jar of water. So he ate and drank, and lay down again. And the angel of the Lord came back the second time, and touched him, and said, "Arise and eat, because the journey is too great for you." So he arose, and ate and drank; and went in the strength of that food forty days and forty nights as far as Horeb, the mountain of God.

1 Kings 19:5-8

Elijah didn't want to eat. He fasted due to an overwhelming situation, but this was actually a demonstration that he was not taking care of himself. An angel continued to prompt him to eat. A very good example that sometimes it is not healthy to fast, and if the Holy Spirit prompts you to eat—eat!

Another purpose for fasting is to set the body free from ungodly attachments or indulgences in food. God has truly blessed us with abundance of food from this earth, but "if not kept in check by periodic abstinence, food can lure our hearts into worshipping the stomach."[22]

We should live soberly and see food as a gift from above, given for the purpose of growing in oneness with Him. Fasting/detoxing is a powerful tool for health, cleansing, corporate strength and spiritual empowerment, and will bless your life with the gift of health, healing, and renewed vitality.[7]

It is not advisable to take on a total fast as we are too toxic and mineral deficient today. Any twenty-one day fast should not be attempted without supervision by a licensed health care provider. The following are some guidelines for fasting:[21]

1. Fast as you can, not as you can't. Not everyone is capable of omitting all foods even for a few hours especially if you are pregnant, nursing, young, or elderly. Try limiting certain foods or meals.

2. Choose a course and stick with it. Traditional fasts are centered around such holidays as Easter. However, another option might be to choose one or two days a week and maintain the discipline all year.

3. Remember that fasting is not a matter of law but the choice of the heart.

4. Feast at appropriate times. To be truly effective, feasting after a fast should be gradual. But a feast can be used as a celebratory function after fasting to enjoy the bounty of creation.

5. For more detailed juice fasting recipes, I highly recommend, *Toxic Relief*, by Don Colbert M.D.

6. Those with certain medical conditions should not fast at all without medical supervision.

Drainage

Another way to improve our health is through drainage. **Drainage** is the process of ensuring the elimination channels are functioning optimally.[21] The elimination channels are the bladder, bowels, skin, tears, lymphs, lungs, and circulation. Drainage starts with adequate water intake. We are attempting to "flush the pipes" and open up the elimination channels. Water requirements are increased when detoxing or undertaking a drainage program. At least 10-12 cups daily during the cleanse is recommended.

Drainage also includes deep breathing. Homeopathic remedies are known to be helpful in this process as well.

Improving our health may not require dramatic changes. It may take discipline and time, but even one action from the above suggestions will improve your health. The health of thousands in our past history was greatly improved because of fasting and detoxification programs and obedience to God.

7

. . . . . .

What Shall We Eat?

The Basics

Carbohydrates

Carbohydrates provide energy, fiber, vitamins and minerals and come from fruit, vegetables, and whole grains. There are "good" carbs and "bad" carbs. The good, or healthy carbohydrates, are unrefined plant foods. These foods provide the vitamins, minerals fiber and other nutrients that are beneficial. The bad carbs are generally regarded as the refined plant foods that have little nutrient value due to the processing involved. These can be categorized as breads, cakes, pies, cereals, noodles, crackers, chips, etc.

A word about grains. It is reported that grains of wheat and barley were first cultivated in 7,000 BC. Corn and rice followed 2,500 years later in 4,500 BC.[25] Grains today are not what they used to be. The grains cultivated back in ancient times and with our European ancestors were truly whole grain with all nutrients intact, without pesticides or herbicides. The people conducted extreme lengths to process their grain to remove the phytic acid and other grain toxins. Their process consisted of the following:

- Pure, rich, uncontaminated soil
- Careful grain harvesting, including slow drying in the sun

- Aging and fermenting the grains
- Storing the grains carefully, with the outer hull to preserve freshness
- Grinding the grains fresh before preparation
- Combining grains with other foods such as dairy
- Generally removing the bran and germ from the grain
- Using starters in low phytase grains.[29]

The people of those times also developed certain biology to adapt to the foods that were available. Our bodies today are not physiologically designed to eat grains in their raw form. In the last hundred years or more, farmed grains are grown with pesticides and herbicides. The residues stay on the surface of the foods and are absorbed into the foods as well. Animals graze on this food. In the process of stripping the grains of their important nutrients, enhancing the look and texture of the flours, chemical additives are added. Synthetic vitamins are added back in. Generally the grains are not sprouted and are heat treated.

Now, due to modern farming practices, we don't go to the same lengths of removing the phytic acids and have to predigest the grains through the process of fermentation and then cooking. In the absence of careful grain preparation including fermentation, a host of diseases appear.[29] We are seeing one fall-out of this grain adulteration—Celiac Disease and gluten intolerance, or corn sensitivities. According to Dr. Hyman in his article, "Gluten, What You Don't Know may be Killing You," there has been a 400 percent increase in celiac in the last 50 years.

The overconsumption of high-carbohydrate grain-based foods such as bran, fibrous breakfast cereals, whole-wheat bread, all contain high amounts of phytates (which block minerals) and can actually lead to intestinal problems, osteoporosis, and increased weight. Dr. Mellanby concluded that most cereals (and this includes whole grain) contain toxic substances that can affect the nervous system. Consuming grains can lead to B vitamin deficiencies, tooth decay, and a variety of other diseases.[29] He also advises to avoid sprouted corn and corn in general due to the genetically modified (GMO) process of corn. Animals know what is right for them to eat and typically will not eat GMO corn unless forced to do so. Animals that have been forced to eat this GMO corn have had reproductive problems.[29]

Fats

Fats provide energy and insulation, nourishes and strengthens cell membranes, controls inflammation, and comes from cold-pressed olive oil, cod liver oil, fish, sunflower oil, sesame oil, flaxseed oil, walnut oil, coconut oil, raw nuts, butter, avocado, tallow, lard, and seeds.

The good fats are EPA/DHA/GLA/ALA. Cod liver oil, grape seed oil, walnut oil, flaxseed oil, and olive oil are rich in EPA and DHA. These promote healthy cholesterol levels and maintain healthy brain and nerve tissue function. Any Essential Fatty Acid should be fresh, not heated, no solvents used to extract the oil, and should be kept cool.

The "bad" fats are the hydrogenated oils or partially hydrogenated or fractionated. Trans-fats, as they are referred, come from adding hydrogen to vegetable oil through hydrogenation to extend shelf life. These are the heart clogging oils and are industrially processed liquid oils. Trans-fat oils are found in mayonnaise, margarine, commercial salad oils, breads, cakes, and cookies. Corn oil, canola, and safflower oils are typically highly rancid due to being processed with high heat and chemical solvents. The clear bottles for packaging allow for light to further degrade and oxidize them. Liquid oils should be packaged in dark glass bottles to block out light. Always refrigerate them when not in use for longer storage life. The immune, cardiovascular, and digestive systems are damaged by these partially rancid cooking oils.

Although canola oil is recognized as a "healthy" oil it is far from healthy. Canola oil is made from something called rapeseed. Rapeseed actually had to be bred over the years to reduce the percentage of a problematic component of rapeseed, called erucic acid.[15] It comes from the name, Canadian Oil. Commercial grade Canola oil has shown trans levels of fat as high as 4.6%. It is typically extracted and refined using high heat, pressure, and petroleum solvents such as hexane. Most canola oil undergoes a process of caustic refining, degumming, bleaching, and deodorization, all using high heat and questionable chemicals. The processing and oxidation of the polyunsaturated component of canola oil, is what makes it unhealthy for human consumption, and is highly unstable under heat, light, and pressure. This heavily oxidizes the polyunsaturates which increases free radicals in your body. The end result of all of this refining and processing are oils that are highly inflammatory in your body when you ingest them, potentially contributing to heart disease, weight gain, and other degenerative diseases.[15] This rancid oil has no health benefits.[29]

While mainstream media likes to demonize "saturated" fats, these fats have health benefits that have sustained us for thousands of years. These fats are in butter, raw milk, meat fats, and coconut oil and carry fat-soluble vitamins A, D, and K. They provide integrity to cell walls and promote the body's use of essential fatty acids. These fats (when consumed in small quantities and in moderation and correctly) do not cause heart disease, rather it is the oxidized trans-fats that leads to stiff cell walls that contribute to this disease. Saturated fats also strengthen the immune and nervous system as well as suppress inflammation.[35] Butter alone contains other nutrients such as lecithin, a natural fat emulsifier, iodine, chromium, zinc, manganese, and selenium. Over half the fat in the brain is saturated. If we take away saturated fats, what would happen to our brain function? According to Weston A. Price, low-fat diets have been linked to failure to thrive in children, yet low-fat diets are recommended for school aged children.

Protein

Protein builds and repairs cell growth, provides enzymes, neurotransmitters, and hormones necessary for muscles. Protein comes from beans and rice, nuts, tofu, Hemp hearts, chicken, fish, turkey, beef, and lamb.

Protein is an important nutrient but many people over consume poor quality protein in the form of bacon, steak, and sausage which can lead to inflammation and waste buildup. The body needs .8 grams per body weight, or a person's weight times .0469 which equals the amount of ounces of protein needed with a meal. Athletes need far more than this. According to the research by K.C. Craichy, the literature suggests that the range of protein requirements are between .5 and 100 percent of body weight in grams and the mid to upper levels of this range are best because most people under consume quality protein.

Animal proteins that are not digested properly release toxic by-products into our bodies. In healthy bodies, the enzymes of the digestive tract neutralize most of these toxins. In former times, the animals raised for food were grass-fed and free ranged meaning they freely roamed around the area of land where they were raised. There were no crowded stock yards and chemicals fed to the animals. There were no "factory farms."

In contrast to today's meats and eggs, factory-farmed meats and eggs promote a profit-driven system of disease in which animal are misused and mistreated. Air and the environment are polluted from the cesspools of these factories. The animals are confined to small corrals, loaded with chemicals to keep them alive, and hormones to speed growth. Their diet is not their natural diet. Added to this the packaged lunch meats consumed contain many harmful food additives such as BHT, nitrates, and sodium benzoate.

Daniel's refusal in 1 Kings to avoid the King's rich food is wisdom to today's adulterated meats and eggs. Choose fresh grass-fed meats and organic eggs whenever possible, and avoid packaged lunch meats with additives altogether.

Calcium

Calcium- If you know anatomy and physiology, you know that good solid bones contribute a great deal to the health and well-being of our physical bodies. Calcium builds strong bones and also transmits nerve impulses, muscle movement, and activates blood coagulation. Seventy percent of bone is calcium. But calcium is not the only element needed for strong bones. Most calcium supplements, such as calcium carbonate, are not usable in the body and ingesting this kind can lead to harm. When we ingest something that is harmful the body launches an attack which can lead to inflammation. Your body works in concert, therefore, in order for calcium to work it needs cofactors like magnesium, potassium, phosphorus, silicone, manganese, vitamin D, and boron, and vitamin K. However, too much phosphorus from excess milk and soda consumption can upset the acid/alkaline (pH) balance of the body. This causes the body to leach calcium from the bones to balance the body's pH.[10] The best sources of calcium are from greens, spinach, kale (in moderation), broccoli, seeds, and nuts. Having proper acid levels in the stomach also contributes to calcium absorption.

Fiber

Fiber regulates blood sugar and bowel peristalsis, binds toxins in the bile, and binds excess estrogens. Sources include beans, grains, vegetables such as broccoli, celery, lettuce, sprouted seeds, and fruits with edible skins. There is twice as much fiber in fruits and four to five times as much in non-starchy vegetables as whole grains.[9]

Although rare, too much fiber can cause other health problems such as intestinal blockage. The body cannot digest fiber. It passes through the intestines in its original, bulky form without being broken down. This is the way our bodies were created. However, by eating too much fiber in the way of breads, bran, brownies, toaster pastries, granola bars, and cereal, this system can backfire. Constipation, cramping and physical blockages within the digestive tract can occur. Drinking lots of water when eating fiber prevents complications such as blockages and constipation.

Vitamins and minerals

Vitamins and minerals -The USDA would have the public believe that all they need to do is follow the Food Guide Pyramid and they'll meet the nutritional requirements the body needs. To maintain health daily our bodies need vitamins (A, B1,B2, B3, B5, B6, B12, C, D, E, K), and minerals (calcium, iron, magnesium, phosphorus, potassium, manganese, sulfur, cobalt, zinc, copper, selenium, iodine, fluorine, germanium, molybdenum, nickel, silicon, sodium, vanadium, boron, and chromium) amino acids from protein (arginine, lysine, histidine, phenylalanine, tyrosine, leucine, isoleucine, methionine, valine, alanine, glycine, proline, glutamic acid, serine, threonine, aspartic acid, tryptophan, cysteine).[21] The value of having individualized nutrition services is to find bioavailable multivitamin supplements, accurate for each persons' unique metabolism, that contain a complete balance of these nutrients rather than taking individual vitamins and minerals in isolation.

God's Design for Food

1.   To sustain us

The Old and New Testament assures us of God's provision. If He feeds the birds of the air and cattle of the field, He will feed us.

He made him ride in the heights of the earth, that he might eat the produce of the fields; he made him to draw honey from the rock, and oil from the flinty rock; Curds (butter) from the cattle, and milk of flock, with fat of lambs, and rams of the breed of Bashan, and goats, with the choicest wheat; and you drank wine, the blood of the grapes.
                                        Deuteronomy 32:13-14

You cause grass to grow for the cattle. You cause plants to grow for people to use. You allow them to produce food from the earth..... and bread to give them strength.
                                        Psalm 104:14-15 (NLT)

And they said to him, "We have here only five loaves, and two fish." He said, "Bring them here to me." Then he commanded the multitudes to sit down on the grass. And He took the five loaves and the two fish, and looking up to heaven, He blessed and broke and gave the loaves to the disciples; and the disciples gave to the multitudes.

Matthew 14:17-19

"Therefore I say to you, do not worry about your life, what you will eat, or what you will drink; nor about your body, what you will put on. Is not life more than food and the body more than clothing? Look at the birds of the air, for they neither sow nor reap nor gather into barns; yet your heavenly Father feeds them. Are you not of more value than they?"

Matthew 6:25-26

2. To eat healthy foods

....brought beds, and basins, earthen vessels and wheat, barley and flour, parched grain and beans, lentils and parched seeds, honey and curds, sheep and cheese of herd, for David and the people who were with him to eat. For they said, "The people are hungry and weary and thirsty in the wilderness."

2 Samuel 17:28-29

Then Abigail made haste and took two hundred loaves of bread, two skins of wine, five sheep ready dressed, five seahs (measures) of roasted grain, one hundred clusters of raisins, and two hundred cakes of figs, and loaded them on donkeys.

1 Samuel 25:18

He causes the grass to grow for the cattle and the vegetation for the service of man, that he may bring forth food from the earth, and wine that makes glad the heart of man, oil to make his face shine, and bread which strengthens man's heart.

Psalm 104:14-15

The use of bread as food was made of wheat or barley and usually made in the form of round flat cakes. Other foods listed in these references were beans, lentils, honey, butter, cheese, raisins, figs, and wine.

> *Butter of kine, and milk of sheep....*
>
> Deuteronomy 32:14

Butter usually signified curdled milk in ancient times. In more modern times the milk was placed in a skin-bottle and suspended from poles and swung side to side by the women to make the butter. Butter (raw) has many healthful benefits. According to the Weston A. Price Foundation, raw butter contains vitamin A, D, K_2, E, lecithin, iodine, and selenium. Vitamin A, D, and K_2 are essential for proper absorption of calcium and phosphorus necessary for strong bones and teeth. The iodine in butter is a highly absorbable form and therefore supportive in thyroid health. In addition, butter provides significant amounts of short and medium-chain fatty acids, which support immune function, boosts metabolism and has anti-microbial properties.

Daniel 1:8-17 again reminds us of the choices between rich food versus pure food. He reminds us of the consequences of choosing the former. Daniel refused to eat the King's rich food and chose to remain spiritually pure by eating only pulse (seeds and nuts). Daniel knew the king's table of rich foods would taste wonderful, but chose to obey God's plan for both his nutritional and spiritual needs. In turn, he reaped God's rewards.

> *Then Jacob said, "Swear to me as of this day." So he swore to him, and sold his birthright to Jacob. And Jacob gave Esau bread and stew of lentils; then he did ate and drank, arose, and went his way. Thus Esau despised his birthright.*
>
> Genesis 25:33-34

We see that Esau sold his birthright for a bowl of stew! He was so focused on his stomach's needs that he ignored the future blessings meant for a first-born son which was the authority over the family and a double portion of his father's wealth. Esau's foolishness is a lesson for us today to avoid caving into desires and spiritual shortsightedness. We, too, can be tempted in this same way as we focus on our own hunger desires and appetites instead of what is right for us by God's design. As with all temptations, if we live according to what feels right, or looks good in food because we are focusing on immediate gratification which only yields temporary fulfillment, then we will miss out on God's blessing of good health in our live. Lasting contentment is the result of pleasing God instead of ourselves.[45]

Change takes time; even with adults. You and your family's habits need gradual changing in small increments. It usually takes three months for a child's (and adult's) hormonal system to adjust to the elimination of unhealthy food choices. The brain is the number one organ involved in thinking, hunger, feelings, and behavior. When starved of vital nutrients the brain suffers from malnutrition. Behavior, concentration, and physical ability are then compromised. The most difficult part is overcoming your resistance to change; second, your family's resistance. You can help with this by having your children participate with your efforts by including them in many of the decisions with you and eating the same way your child eats so that they don't feel left out.

3. To refrain from causing others to stumble

Romans 14:13-26 conveys to not cause our brother to stumble. The strong in faith will not eat or drink something that may injure or cause harm to someone else, which is in essence, or tantamount to, destroying what God has built. We are to bear the failings of the weak. If someone who is overweight eats at our table, we wouldn't put soda and doughnuts before them any more than putting wine in front of someone who is struggling with alcoholism. Samson, in Judges 13:24-25, gave in to his weakness leading to his downfall. We can apply this same principle with food. If doughnuts or coke are your downfall and you know this, then apply the principle of self-control.

But the fruit of the Spirit is love, joy, peace, patience, kindness, goodness, faithfulness, gentleness, self-control; against such there is no law.

Galatians 5:22-23 (RSV)

God, the greatest master nutritionist of all times, has given us an all-purpose diet more than 4,000 years ago. In the Garden of Eden, Adam and Eve were sustained with all the vitamins, minerals, amino acids, and essential fatty acids that their bodies required from the foods that God created to sustain them. Do not let the fads, media hype, celebrity endorsements, special interest industries, and fashions of the world become your criteria for eating.

4. **To live by God's dietary guidelines, not the Food Guide Pyramid or counting calories**

The birds and animals know instinctively what to eat and are not guided by calories. (I know I am stretching this, but attempting to make a point.) If God provides for the birds and animals of the field, why do we need to be so obsessed with calculating the number of calories or points to stay healthy? I am quite certain that Hippocrates, Jesus, the disciples, or any other generations of our past ancestors did not count calories or points before they ate their food. They ate to live, rather than lived to eat. We have become a generation of people obsessed with counting calories partly due to media influence. "Calories in equals calories out"does not work for everyone. Every person's metabolism is different. Dr. Leo Galland, M.D. says that what matters most about the calories in any food are the nutrients that accompany them. God's dietary guidelines preserved the Israelite's physical health with vegetables, cheese, milk, meat, grains, and wine. From ancient civilizations to our ancestors of World War II lived without the Food Guide Pyramid. We can too; guided by spiritual discernment and in many cases common sense.

5. To eat "good" carbohydrates

In 2 Samuel, God provided David's people with whole grains such as millet, amaranth, beans, lentils and seeds, honey, cheese. Ezekiel gives further instruction on what foods to eat.

Also take for yourself wheat, barley, beans, lentils, millet, and spelt; put them into one vessel, and make bread of them for yourself...
Ezekiel 4:9

And on the banks, on both sides of the river, there will grow all kinds of trees for food. Their leaves will not wither nor their fruit fail, but they will bear fresh fruit every month, because the water for them flows from the sanctuary. Their fruit will be for food, and their leaves for healing.
Ezekiel 47:12 (RSV)

6. To eat simple

Foods were prepared in as simple and natural way as possible, which is a good guideline for us today. Matthew 3:4 reveals that John's diet, at one time, was as simple as locusts and honey. Food combining, such as eating a meat and potatoes dinner, can lead to digestive problems. Why is this? Proteins require a series of acid digestive juices to digest the protein and a series of alkaline digestive juices to digest the starch in potatoes. Alkaline neutralizes acid and the result is no digestion. The food just sits there....degrading, souring, putrefying. Raw and lightly steamed vegetables, fats with vegetables, or proteins with vegetables are easier on the digestive system.[11]

7. To eat fermented foods

Fermented foods are sauerkraut, cottage cheese, pickles, pickled foods, kombucha, and kefir. Fermented foods provide a natural preservative and protect the food from dangerous organisms. Fermentation is effective in releasing important nutritional compounds through "pre-digestion"that would otherwise pass through the human digestive system undigested and unused. Many fermented drinks are known to relieve intestinal problems.[39]

> *So Abraham hastened into the tent to Sarah and said, "Quickly, make ready three measures of fine meal; knead it and make cakes." And Abraham ran to the herd, took a tender and good calf, gave it to a young man, and he hastened to prepare it. So he took butter and milk and the calf which he had prepared, and set it before them; and he stood by them under the tree as they ate.*
>
> Genesis 18:6-8

Thousands of years ago, Abraham wanted to serve his best meat, dairy, and fermented cream curds to entertain his guests.[39] The practice of fermentation since the earliest times was common as refrigeration was not yet invented. People in ancient times, and until refrigeration was invented, relied on fermented foods. They knew about the value of protection from microbials in food and drinks.

Archeological finds have shown that even during the hunter/ gatherer times, people fermented a plant similar to the cabbage. The Chinese fermented their cabbage in rice wine as far back as 2000 years ago. Emperor Tiberius carried barrels of sauerkraut on his extended journeys in the Middle East. The sauerkraut protected him and his men from intestinal infections. The first instructions on fermentation were written by the roman scholar Pliny in 50 A.D.[61]

Now days with refrigeration we have lacto-fermented foods such as yogurt, kefir, cheeses, cottage cheese, cultured cream, and cultured coconut. These foods inoculate and build the gut flora with beneficial probiotics.

8. To prepare our own food

When you eat the labor of your hands, you shall be happy, and it shall be well with you.

Psalms 128:2

Matthew Henry's commentary of this passage states that an idle life is a miserable, uncomfortable life and that we should not be forced to live upon the labors of other people. It is as much a mercy as a duty, with quietness to work and eat our own bread. They and theirs shall enjoy what they get.

Other suggestions for eating the healthy way:

- Of all the diet books in print, The Zone Diet, The South Beach Diet, Atkins Diet, Eat This, Not That, and others, The Paleolithic diet, as researched by Robb Wolf, appears to be the most closely related to the diet in biblical times. Wolf's research dates back to pre-biblical era as known as the "hunter-gatherer" period. It consists of an abundance of fruits, vegetables, nuts, seeds, seafood, healthy fats, and lean meats.[66] Olive oil, which is full of antioxidants and healthy fat, is the principle source of fat along with flaxseed oil, walnut oil, and butter. Dairy intake is primarily cheese (goat) and yoghurt in low to moderate amounts, and very little fresh milk. The advice is to consume small amounts of lean meat, poultry, and fish. Wine is consumed in small quantities with meals.
- The Mediterranean diet which was consumed by the cultures in Europe, North Africa, and Middle East for thousands of years is characterized by whole grains, large quantities of fruits and vegetables grown locally and consumed in season, eggs, fish, poultry, wine, honey, and olive oil used generously.
- Eat foods that are not rich, greasy and fried, processed or commercially made grain products.
- Many gluten-free grain products are made with brown rice and other high starch flours. Brown rice is very high in phytic acid

and this is toxic in high quantities. White rice has less phytic acid but is also much more refined and low in fiber. These foods will raise blood sugar or can set the stage for another food sensitivity or toxic overload or other health challenges like low iron, vitamin deficiency, or inflammation. Eating rice in combination with vitamin C rich foods like collard greens disables the phytate levels in rice.

- Eat foods in season and according to climate. Pay attention to cause and effect. (Consuming lots of sugar can lead to headache, or overeating can lead to a stomachache).
- Eat a plant based diet, including low phytic acid and low lectin grains such as rice or buckwheat, fruit, vegetables, legumes, nuts, and seeds such as pumpkin, sunflower, or chia.
- Include plenty of fat-soluble foods containing vitamins A and D to the diet, such as pumpkins, yams, tuna, turnips, beet greens, fish (and yes, fish heads), sardines, cod liver oil, eggs, organic butter, and spinach.
- Eat plants that contain antioxidant phytochemicals such as pomegranates, figs, cranberries, blueberries, green leafy vegetables, garlic, and parsley.
- Consume portions of protein throughout the day to balance blood sugar.
- Fruits and vegetables are rich in antioxidants and immune-building nutrients such as beta carotene (vitamin A), lycopene, flavonoids, vitamin C, E, selenium, magnesium and zinc. Leafy greens (lettuce, kale, spinach), carrots, bell peppers, tomatoes, onions, broccoli and squash are excellent sources of vitamin C, beta carotene and many other naturally occurring antioxidants (also fruits such as citrus, melons, peaches and grapes). Vitamin E, zinc and magnesium are abundant in whole grains, wheat germ, sunflower seeds, almonds and walnuts. Broccoli, fish and eggs are selenium rich foods.
- Avoid all GMO or GE foods such as corn, soy, canola oil, milk, and cottonseed oil.

Improved blood lipids, reduced pain, reduced allergies, balanced energy, stable blood sugars, and improved sleep are some of the many benefits of eating a clean Paleolithic or Mediterranean diet according to Robb Wolf.[6]

What are "Super Foods" and are they Biblical?

Super Foods contain concentrations of nutrients in combination, providing balanced nutritional support. These so called super foods are much more desirable than mega doses of isolated nutrients. Some of these include: Bee Pollen, Blue green algae, Spirulina, Chlorella, Marine Phytoplankton, Evening primrose oil, Borage oil, Black current oil, Flaxseed oil, Kelp, Wheat germ oil, and Brewer's Yeast.

Though biblical references were not located for most of these foods, bee pollen is referenced in scripture as "honey" on numerous occasions. Chlorella contains chlorophyll, which is in all green plants, so it would have been richly supplied in the natural plant diet throughout history. Kelp and phytoplankton come from the sea and seafood has been a main staple in the Middle East since ancient times.

Now the flax and the barley were struck, for the barley was in the head, and the flax was in bud.

Exodus 9:31

Flax, found in several scriptural references, was grown extensively in Egypt, and linen in those days was derived from flax. The seeds were used medicinally as a demulcent, emollient, and laxative. We know now that flaxseeds contain a source of omega 3 oils, alpha-linolenic acid, dietary fiber, and lignans.

Everything in Moderation

While there are an abundance of food choices available today, scripture admonishes moderation and self-discipline, and caution for all of us.

Do not mix with winebibbers (heavy drinkers of wine), or with gluttonous eaters of meat; For the drunkard and the glutton will come to poverty, and drowsiness will clothe a man with rags.

Proverbs 23:20-21

...that the older men be sober, grave, temperate, sound in faith, in charity, in patience.

Titus 2:2

All things are lawful for me, but all things are not helpful.

1 Corinthians 6:12

God created us with legitimate appetites for food, and He has indicated throughout scriptures that too much of anything is detrimental to the body, mind, or spirit. Self-control is listed as spiritual fruit. God gives us the strength and wisdom to remain within the boundaries He has set for an abundance of desires.[47]

True temperance includes moderation in things good for us as well as abstinence in things harmful. As in 1 Corinthians 6:12 reminds us, just because it is food and available to eat, doesn't mean it is beneficial for us to eat. We cannot use the statement of "Everything in Moderation" to justify our poor choices. Many things in life are terribly destructive even in moderation: cigarettes, drugs, idolatry, jealousy, etc.

By being temperate, we are preserving our health. Too much of one thing is harmful. Too much sunshine, too much exercise, too much sugar, too much food, too much worry, too much T.V., too much coffee, etc. "Those who can't say no to their own desires end up enslaved to them." -Charles Stanley, 2012

Eat the right amount, the right foods, and at the right time.

Our physical health is maintained by what we eat and what we put into our body, and affects all of our organs and tissues. One might think, "God doesn't care about what I eat." Yes, He does. What fuels the Temple? Would we put kerosene in our car to make it move? A wrong diet, or an indulged appetite of a good one, greatly hinders mental and physical efficiency, injures our bodies, and keeps our minds from functioning as well as they should.[11]

But I eat healthy! Why am I still sick?

This question is under the assumption that if you eat healthy you won't get sick. By whose standard are you measuring yourself that you are eating healthy? The Food Guide Pyramid? The RDA? Your doctor? Your child's school lunch menu? Your friends? Mainstream medical and media would have you believe that if you just eat right and exercise that your health problems will all go away. You read good books, eat vegetables, only drink one cup of coffee and can't understand why you are sick.

First, we live in a fallen world. You've read in the previous chapters about how we have become so disordered. We can eat what we think are the right foods, but we have to contend with air pollution, contaminated soil and contaminated foods even if labeled organic.

Second, what is eating healthy? Media would have you believe that non-fat, low-fat, microwaved, deep fried, cereal, milk and orange juice for breakfast are healthy. Oatmeal may be relatively healthy, but if you are eating a Genetically Modified brand, it is not healthy. Eating a prepackaged meal may look healthy with just the right amount of protein, carb, and fat content, but that food was already cooked once. So it is not fresh food and then it is microwaved to heat it up a second time which leaves the nutrient value questionable at best. All processed food is high in sodium. Thinking that eating canned soup is just as nutritious as fresh vegetable soup is also misguided. After ten years in business reading hundreds of food intake journals, I have seen people's perception of healthy is greatly misinformed.

Third, drinking juice over fresh fruits. Juice is healthier than soda, but they are also concentrated sources of sugar with empty calories. Juices can also be laced with hidden flavors and added colorings.

Fourth, allergens and cross reactants. Food, as healthy as it may appear may be poison to one person and life to another. You may have an unrecognized food sensitivity to a relatively unsuspecting food. Some common food sensitivities are wheat, corn, dairy, soy, eggs, shellfish, chocolate, and nuts. But so are broccoli, asparagus, tomatoes, tangerines, or spinach to someone else. If your body can't process certain foods, this will lead to inflammation which can bring on illness. Get tested to find out your food sensitivities.

Fifth, cheating. Many health coaches or trainers say you can have one cheat day. Who are you really cheating? And what are you cheating with? Sugar? Coffee? Bread? If you are a sugar addict and go all week without sugar and load up on sugar on your "cheat" day, you are undoing what you've just done for five days, and it will take your body another two to three days to recover from your cheat day. How productive is that? It also just prolongs the addiction to that food item. I wouldn't any more tell an alcoholic, "It's okay." "You've been a good guy all week, you can cheat on one day." It may sound like a ridiculous comparison, but the theory behind it not any different.

Sixth, over heating those veggies cooks the nutrient benefit right out of them. Or eating left-overs. People love left-overs. They say it saves in preparation time. If the nutrients were cooked out the day before, reheating further degrades the nutrients. Left-overs can weaken digestion, cause toxins, and are low in 'life force.' If used regularly, these foods could contribute to a number digestive diseases including irritable bowel syndrome (IBS) and the like. There seems to be a difference between what food scientists call spoilage bacteria and pathogens. Spoilage bacteria form into slimy films on lunch meat, soggy edges on vegetables or stinky chicken. But the pathogens that do make you sick are odorless, colorless and invisible. Since consumers can't count on looks or smell, instead use the rule of four: no more than four days at 40 degrees Fahrenheit or 4 degrees centigrade. Although I prefer to only use one day and none after that. Freezing fresh food at zero degree Fahrenheit will keep it safe indefinitely. Other factors that can increase risk for illness include:

- Double-dipping will make food go bad faster because it transfers saliva into the food, which promotes bacterial growth. One study even found that three to six double dips transferred about 10,000 bacteria from an eater's mouth to the dip sample.

This also applies to sharing eating utensils with someone else who may be infected with a pathogen.

- Putting leftovers away in a big clump may also promote food spoilage. This is because the food at the center of the mass will take longer to cool, which means bacteria will continue to grow even after it's in the refrigerator.
- Vegetable oils, such as those in mayonnaise and salad dressing, break down over time and turn rancid. Though you may not notice this change the rancid oils can cause damage in your body.
- If you leave leftovers or any food out too long, it will speed spoilage. Two hours is generally the maximum they should be left out, though the sooner you refrigerate them the better (remember to factor in the time it takes to drive back from the grocery store, and the time it takes you to unpack your groceries).

Seventh, counting calories. "It's only 50 calories, so it must be healthy." The food may only have 50 calories, but if it is packaged, or processed it is loaded with unhealthy sodium and preservatives. You don't need to count calories if you are eating real food.

Eighth, eating 100% raw or vegan. This is a myth to think that eating this way is the healthiest. Weston A. Price in his research disproved this. Illness follows if you are missing valuable nutrients not found in 100% raw foods.

Ninth, lean cuts of meat. The leanest cuts of meat may have the highest sodium levels. Since lean meats are less juicy, manufacturers enhance turkey, chicken and beef products by pumping them full of a liquid solution that contains water and salt leading to excess sodium intake. Stick with grass-fed beef and organic free range chicken and turkey.

Tenth, poor food combining. Proper food combining ensures that everything you eat stands the best chance of digesting. Its purpose is to make digestion easier. The most common mistake people make are combining a protein like a meat with a starch such as a potato. Think about all those happy meal hamburgers, hotdogs, and steak and potato meals. This combination just doesn't digest. It takes acid digestive juices to digest the protein and alkaline juices to digest the starch. Alkaline neutralizes acid, so no digestion happens. When food doesn't digest, it rots. You may think you are eating healthy, but the combination of the food may be your culprit. Good guidelines for proper combining are proteins with vegetables and vegetables with starches. Fruits do not combine well with protein or starches either. Eat fruit alone.

Lastly, it may not be what you are eating. Cortisol imbalance, digestion and malabsorption issues from hidden microbials, electropollution from cell phones and Wi-Fi, fluorescent lights, Interference Fields from past surgeries or trauma are some other factors to consider.

Health is not just about eating healthy. There are so many variables from which to consider. Although not always is it God's will to heal people of their illness in spite of how well a person eats and drinks, He allows suffering for a reason; either to experience His comfort, to grow in hope, holiness, or faith, or to procure our attention about something in our life. It is our call to place our trust for whatever outcome He allows, and pray for God's ultimate will and healing plan, while still obeying the physical laws He set in place many years ago. As Gideon found out in the book of Judges Chapter 6, God never abandons us. In times of temptation, danger, or difficulty He will never leave us and will guide us in the trials we face.

8

. . . . . .

Is it Okay to Eat Pig and Seafood?

Pigs

Pigs eat anything they find including their own young if they are stressed, sick or if dead pigs or other animals are in the same pen. They eat cancers off themselves or other pigs. They eat excretions of other animals in the same feed lots.

The pig's digestive tract digests ingested material in four hours or less, causing their tissues to contain high levels of fat and toxins. Pigs have little to no sweat glands so they retain more toxins in their tissues. They roll in the mud to keep cool. Pigs contain 19 different types of worms including Trichinella Spiralis, a type of roundworm that causes Trichinosis.[67]

Modern farming and feeding practices have cut down on the occurrence of tapeworms, but overcrowding on farms can also increase the risk of viral diseases. It is apparent from the media that Swine Flu has caused great amount of fear and worry. Swine flu virus does not cause disease, but seeks out an environment where it can thrive —an oxygen depleted or weak immune body. For a pandemic, the flu has to find an environment that favors virulence and ease of transmission such as occurred in 1918 during WW1 on the Western Front.[28]

Pigs and Trichinosis

Twelve cases per year in the United States have been reported from 1997-2001.[15] Trichinosis can cause joint stiffness and pain, which commonly is mistaken for many other diseases such as: heart disease, arthritis, asthma, gout, mumps, and gallbladder disease. Linked to Hepatitis E in the U.S.[69]

Pig Infections and Infestations

Bladder worms are tapeworms in humans. These affect the muscle, diaphragm, heart, brain, eyes and liver. The worms can grow to be 3-6 feet in humans.

Clostridium Profingens or Enteritis Necroticum can cause stomach pain, vomiting of blood and severe lowering of blood pressure.

Porcine Endogenous Retrovirus is found in all pig tissue and may be passed to humans by pig tissue transplants.[59]

Curing, drying, smoking, microwaving, does not consistently kill infective worms which is why the FDA strongly advises to cook all pork thoroughly.[67]

……. and the pig, for though it divides the hoof, thus making a split hoof, it does not chew cud, it is unclean to you. You shall not eat of their flesh nor touch their carcasses; they are unclean to you.
Leviticus 11:7-8 (NASV)

Pork was listed as one of the unclean meats. Now, we don't live under the Levitical Law, but under grace. But remember, this was a health "law" and is relevant today. So, should you eat pig? That decision has to be between you and God, but if you do, I urge you to purchase organic nitrate free ham or pork at a Whole Foods market or Co-op. Most commercial and well known meat packaging companies are not as trustworthy with their treatment of the animals. Support organic farmers and those that use humane treatments with their animals.

Seafood

Old Testament law in Leviticus 11:10 and Deuteronomy 14:9-10 warned not to eat sea scavengers. In 1953 Dr. David Macht, M.D. conducted research in which he tested every clean and unclean food listed in Deuteronomy 14 and Leviticus 11. He found that every single type of meat that was listed in scripture as unclean tested highly toxic. Every meat that was allowed by scripture was non-toxic. He and his team of researchers found that this was true 100% of the time. (*Bulletin of the History of Medicine, Johns Hopkins School of Medicine*)

> *"But all in the seas or in the rivers that do not have fins and scales, all that move in the water or any living thing which is in the water, they are an abomination to you."*
>
> Leviticus 11:10

> *These you may eat of all that are in the waters: you may eat all that have fins and scales. And whatever does not have fins and scales you shall not eat; it is unclean for you.*
>
> Deuteronomy 14:9-10

Environmental scientists are finding that shrimp, crab, lobster and oysters are becoming dangerously toxic today with mercury and other heavy metals. Even farmed fish can contain varying amounts of toxins from DDT to pesticides.

Although Hebrew Law of purity forbade these foods for their association with cultural practices, there is evidence they were onto something important that long ago. Mounting evidence of mercury is showing up in seafood, and shellfish allergies are increasing, which is another good reason to avoid certain seafood such as shell-fish, shell-fish oils such as krill oil and green lipped muscle oil, and partake in a detoxification program.

On the other hand, since God did create seafood for us to eat there must be something healthy about these foods. Fish have many beneficial properties. Fish are rich in protein, potassium, vitamins, minerals, and essential omega-3 fats. Protecting the arteries from damage, inhibiting blood clots, reducing blood triglycerides, easing symptoms of rheumatoid arthritis, fighting inflammation, and helping to regulate the immune system are other benefits of fish.[39] Sardines alone provide three times more calcium and phosphorus than milk and as much protein as steak. They contain high amounts of DHA and EPA fat, CoQ10, vitamin B12, selenium and vitamin D, and as long as we have a healthy functioning immune system and adequate detoxification system, the toxicities from fish may not totally present a problem. It is better to ingest the fish to get the omega -3's than to go without.

9

. . . . . .

What Shall We Drink?

In my quest for liquids that were consumed in biblical times only four were found that were common; water, milk, grape juice, and wine.

So he took butter and milk and the calf which he had prepared, and set it before them....

Genesis 18:8

Ho, everyone who thirsts, come to the waters; and he who has no money, come, buy and eat! Come, buy wine and milk without money and without price.

Isaiah 55:1(RSV)

When the wine failed, the mother of Jesus said to him, "They have no wine."

John 2:3-11(RSV)

Water

The world's first civilizations were built near rivers. These people knew the importance of water for themselves, their animals, and their crops. Their water systems were technological advances of their time.

Our body is 70% water. Every cell inside of us is constantly being bathed in water. Water removes toxins, nourishes and bathes cells, helps convert food to energy, cushions joints, balances electrolytes. Water in the blood brings nutrition and oxygen to our tissues, and carries off wastes. Water is the central regulator of energy and osmotic balance in the body, and is the main solvent for all foods, vitamins, and minerals. It is used in the breakdown of food into smaller particles and their eventual metabolism and assimilation.[2] If injury occurs, coagulants come out of the fluid and stop the bleeding, while white blood cells emerge from the blood stream and begin attacking poisonous substance. Without enough water this process is hindered.

Our brain 85% water.[21] Adequate intake of water is absolutely essential. We were designed to consume adequate amounts of pure water. The past 100 years water has been replaced with soda, coffee, tea, juice, energy drinks, and other caffeinated liquids. These liquids cause dehydration. Dehydration has been linked to heartburn, angina, arthritis, back pain, cancer, kidney stones, and colitis. The body can show deep dehydration without a dry mouth. A dry mouth is one of the very last indicators of dehydration, and by that time, many other functions of the body have already been shut down.[2] If our brain doesn't get the volume of water it needs, the body will take water from joints, spinal discs and even organs in order to supply the brain.

Water Everywhere and not a Drop to Drink

More than two-thirds of the earth's surface is covered with water and yet we are at a point in our history when pure water is almost impossible to find. Recent US government studies show that approximately 1 person in 5 in the US drinks contaminated water sources.[21] This means that there are alarming levels of DDT and other pesticides, heavy metals and other environmental toxins such as, PCBs or dioxins in water; even bottled water.[2]

Healthy Water

Drink water from your own cistern, flowing water from your own well.

Proverbs 5:15(RSV)

Proverbs 5:15-18 conveys the idea that the only water source we could trust as being clean was our own well. I think that is wisdom for us today! Pure, healthy water is "hard," containing minerals and slightly alkaline pH. The more alkaline the body is, the less chance of disease.[2] Disease thrives on an acidic internal environment. Increasing the intake of vegetables and fruits increases the amount of water consumed as these foods are as much as 70% water. Reverse osmosis and filtered are also excellent choices for water.

Distilled water is thought of as the best water to drink. Actually, this is not advisable as it can interfere with electrolyte balance.

How much water should a person consume? Take one's weight and divide by two equals about how many ounces of water a person should consume daily, especially when detoxing or heavily exercising. Of course, in hotter weather and vigorous exercise it may require more. It is important to maintain water balance because if not, blood can thicken and flow with greater difficulty, and can cause stress to a heart that has to pump this sludged blood. Drink water before and after meals, and at room temperature to ensure proper enzyme and digestion function. Too hot or too cold interferes with digestion. Drinking 2-3 glasses of water first thing in the morning also helps to activate and hydrate internal organs.

Fluoridation

Dr. Dean Burk-former researcher with the National Cancer Institute found that one tenth of all cancer deaths in the US could be linked to fluoridation of our water.[2] Dr. Burk also believes that fluoride is a major carcinogen and responsible for tens of thousands of deaths per year and that stopping fluoride will reduce cancer deaths. He continues to state that as early as 1952 there was evidence that fluoride shortened life span of mice from cancer and that people in fluoridated cities might die of cancer at an early age due to exposure.[3]

After a forty day trial in Illinois over the use of fluoride in their water, Judge Ronald A. Newman decided that there was no evidence to support the notion that fluoridation is a safe effective means to support dental health.[2]

Fluoridation has been linked to birth defects, allergies, fatigue, headaches, urinary tract irritations and genetic damage to plants and animals.

Again, fluoride was not used in water thousands of years ago. Peoples' teeth were not suffering from lack of fluoride.

Chlorination

Dr. James Price, M.D. published a book in the late 1960s on the relationship between treated water and degenerative diseases. He concluded that "nothing can negate the basic cause of arthrosclerosis, heart attack and most common forms of stroke as being the chlorine contained in our drinking water."[20] Chlorine also has the ability to damage the intestinal flora leading to a host of gastrointestinal disorders.

Through bathing, showering, and swimming we are exposed to high amounts of chlorine as well as toluene, ethyl-benzene and styrene.

Those who swim do get a larger exposure to chlorine; however, one has to weigh the benefits of the exercise as opposed to the damages of the exposure. Showering afterwards thoroughly with non-chlorinated water or using a shower filter is helpful at reducing exposure.

Randall Fitzgerald cautions that chlorine is a chemical with the ability to transform other chemicals into mimics of estrogen, the female hormone, and those who drink chlorinated water are at a higher risk of developing breast cancer.[12]

Milk

Curds from the cattle, and milk of the flock, with fat of lambs; and rams of the breed of Bashan, and goats, with the choicest wheat.....

Deuteronomy 32:14

"And carry these ten cheeses to the captain of their thousand, and see how your brothers fare, and bring back news of them."

1 Samuel 17:18

....honey and curds, sheep and cheese of the herd, for David and the people who were with him to eat.

2 Samuel 17:29a

......Who plants a vineyard, and does not eat of its fruit? Or who tends a flock and does not drink of the milk of the flock?

1 Corinthians 9:7b

These passages above show the kinds of milk, and milk products, and other liquids consumed by God's people. Cow's milk and goat's milk were commonplace. Milk and grape juice were common in the New Testament as well.

Today's Milk consists of Cow's milk, Raw milk, Almond, Rice milk, Soy milk, Similac, and all varieties of 1%, 2%, low-fat, non-fat, and skim.

The Lord describes the land of promise as the land flowing with milk and honey. Today, America could be referred to as the land of soda and chips. However, USDA reports that Americans consumed an average of 1.8 cups of dairy per person, per day in 2005, and drink an average of 56 gallons of soda per person, per year. So in spite of the high soda consumption, Americans still consume milk..... thinking that it is doing their body good. It is not surprising with all the cute milk ads displaying happy cows, beautiful women with milk mustaches influencing consumers into believing that milk does their "body good."

Is this milk the same milk that was consumed thousands of years ago or even a hundred years ago? Not in the least. Today's milk is altered, stripped, and reconstituted leaving it no longer the pure viable nutritious or even healthy product it used to be. With all the processing and additives involved guarantees that a person will be consuming a mixture of substances from all over the country, not just from the one cow it originally came from.[52]

The subject of adult humans consuming cow's milk today is a very controversial one. On one hand many scientific studies have linked milk intake with: intestinal colic-irritation-bleeding, anemia, allergies and Salmonella infections in infants, Bovine Leukemia Virus, and childhood diabetes, arteriosclerosis, high cholesterol, as well as many other disorders. A half liter of milk consumed daily increases risk of diabetes three times.[38] In addition, dairy by its nature is acidifying inside the body. To counter this, the body will draw on its acid buffer mineral, calcium, from the bones. As calcium is extracted to neutralize the acid, our bones become weak. Unless a person has calcium reserves in their liver from food or proper supplementation, the body will pull calcium from the bones to compensate for the lack of alkalizing minerals. Osteoporosis is the fall out of this action. It is best to consume calcium rich foods instead of relying on milk solely for calcium support.

Is it truly possible that a food that has nurtured man since the biblical times has suddenly become harmful to him? Should we blame the cow? If a deficient plant produces deficient food, is it reasonable to assume that this could lead to nutrient deficient humans? The same could be said of cow's milk. If a cow is deficient of nutrients, then the milk could be deficient, which could cause the human's metabolism to react in some manner.[36] As Pottenger points out, "Cholesterol is not the villain; the villain is what man does to his cattle and milk."[36]

How it is that milk is not what it used to be? It's called Food Politics. Media deception. Money. From ancient civilizations up to even one hundred years ago milk went from the cow to the table and provided healthy proteins, enzymes, calcium, and vitamins. The process from cow to table now involves many steps. One step is homogenization which is the process of passing it at high speeds through very small holes to create a uniform texture and prevent the cream from separating and rising to the top. This high pressure smashes the milk molecules so hard that it splits and exposes the molecules to oxygen. When molecules are exposed to oxygen the fats become oxidized. According to Kristin Wartman and other research studies, it is the oxidized cholesterol that raises the LDL.[52]

Oxidized fats are the main culprit for high cholesterol, atherosclerosis, and high LDL. This damaged cholesterol is much different than the good cholesterol that is found in eggs, butter and whole or raw milk. These foods raise HDL.

In addition, milk is pasteurized, heated to at least 145 degrees. The CDC continues to mandate all milk to be pasteurized because they claim raw milk is "150 times more dangerous" due to the bacteria than pasteurized milk."[1] This destruction of bacteria in milk by heat processing is assumed to be essential in preventing disease because of the findings of Louis Pasteur's studies. However, according to Pottenger's studies, the good properties of milk are affected by the heat processing and the entire physiochemical state of the milk is altered. Colloids are precipitated and mineral salts are thrown out. Consequently, minerals are rendered less soluble. The antibodies in milk giving immunity to disease are also affected.[36] Pasteurization destroys all enzymes, growth factors and vitamins which make milk very difficult to digest, and can lead to lactose intolerance and other intestinal disorders. According to Francis Pottenger in his studies with cats, which proved similar effects with humans, cooked milk gave the cats various allergies and symptoms of sneezing, wheezing and skin scratching. They were also more irritable and nervous than those who consumed raw or unheated milk.[36]

Up to 32 percent of available calcium is destroyed when food is heated above 150 degrees F.[20] Consequently, this pasteurized milk is a limited source of calcium. In some states, non-fat milk solids are added to the milk in order to thicken it and give it a better mouth feel. Synthetic vitamin A and D are added. So contrary to popular belief that you need milk for vitamins, the body does not absorb synthetic vitamins well. Americans drink skim milk or low-fat milk due to the media frenzy alerting consumers that whole milk will make them fat, on the other hand they are consuming more milk fat in the form of ice cream and half and half with their coffee and then they wonder why their cholesterol levels are so high.

Milk has been found to have 80-200 toxins, hormones, antibiotics, pesticides, sugar, etc. CBS evening news recently reported that seventeen antibiotics are given to cows, but only six of these are tested in milk. The excess hormones can contribute to estrogen dominance and weight gain. It can increase risk of gluten allergies.[38] "Pasteurized, homogenized milk also promotes heart disease, obesity, autoimmune disorders, constipation, sinus congestion and many other chronic health conditions," says Adams. Adams points out that "Pasteurized dairy is produced in the dirtiest milk factories imaginable, where blood, pus, e.coli and other truly dangerous pathogens are routinely bottled into milk containers and fed to consumers." He continues, "The whole point of pasteurization, you see is to kill everything that might be alive in their {the dairy industry} ultra-dirty milk." "The real purpose of pasteurization is not to simply "make milk safe" as is claimed by the CDC, but rather to allow the dairy industry to operate dirty!" As Adams continues, "It's so much easier to just cook the crap out of the milk (yes, there's fecal matter in it) than to clean up their operations, get it?"[1] This again is an example of deception. Thinking that milk is safe just because it is pasteurized is deception garnered by the dairy industry.

Raw milk, on the other hand, is non-pasteurized, from animals that eat fresh grass and other fodder. Raw milk from a reputable dairy operation such as Organic Pastures is the cleanest milk on the planet. It has friendly bacteria in it; the bacteria that is good for you. It's called probiotics.[1] Raw milk has all of the nutrients of protein, fats, hormones, and enzymes needed to digest it and be fully assimilated in the body. "These nutrients are essential for the optimum growth of the human brain as well as the body," remarks Pottenger.[36] Raw milk is very difficult to buy, especially in California. It is best to try to find a farmer that will sell fresh milk directly. If not, use only cultured milk products such as: kefir, whole milk yoghurt, cultured buttermilk, raw cheeses and cultured cream. Grass-fed, or pasture-grazed cow milk is also an alternative.

Is low-fat, nonfat, 2%, or skim milk healthy? Milk is not what it used to be. First of all, milk in biblical times was raw milk, so that is our standard even today. There wasn't a cholesterol or heart disease problem such as what we are experiencing in today's society. Second, there is no such thing as a two percent, low-fat, nonfat, skim milk cow! Period! Again, this is food politics. It is media hype, and dairy industry generated. Third, it goes back to deception. Nonfat milk solids are created through a process of evaporation and high heat drying which removes the moisture from skim milk. Exposure to high heat and oxygen causes fats to oxidize. In low fat or skim milk powdered milk usually is added. And powdered milk contains oxidized fats. According to Michael Pollan, "The low-fat campaign coincided with a dramatic increase in the incidence of obesity and diabetes in America. There is a growing body of evidence that shifting from fats to carbs may lead to weight gain. These refined carbs interfere with insulin metabolism in ways that increase hunger and promote overeating and fat storage in the body."[33] And, to make dairy products low fat, the fat is removed. Then great lengths are taken to preserve the creamy texture by working in all kinds of food additives. That means powdered milk for low-fat or skim milk. Because this milk is now oxidized, the food makers add antioxidants to the milk to compensate; further adulterating the milk. "Removing the fat makes it much harder for your body to absorb the fat-soluble vitamins that are one of the reasons to drink milk in the first place."[33] Blinded to the fact that kid's waistlines are not growing from drinking whole milk, but rather from the fast-food and sugary eating habits, "The Doctors" recommend low-fat milk for children because it has only 100 calories.[51] Dr. Schwartzbein adds, "Eating a low-fat, low-calorie diet over a period of years is one of the surest ways to develop a lifestyle-based endocrine and mood disorder. Hair loss may not be due to a biotin deficiency, it may just mean to get off low-fat foods."[42]

Since the brain is mostly made from fat, you need fats to help your brain produce neurotransmitters, eating healthy fats is essential to mood and a healthy brain. Again, if the milk product is anything other than whole milk, it has been altered from its original state. The body doesn't recognize the foreign or synthetic substances and reacts accordingly by launching an attack. This sets up the cascade of inflammation in the body and can lead to food allergies or other disorders.

Lastly, remember that media and marketing are central in deceiving people into consuming low-fat, or non-fat dairy. Taking a look at nonfat dairy foods such as nonfat cream cheese or nonfat cottage cheese, one will see that it contains neither cream nor cheese. It is processed and should no longer be considered dairy. With all the valuable nutrients stripped, sugars and synthetic vitamins added, diabetes and mood disorders increasing, milk does not "do the body good."

Reasonable Milk Strategies

1. Drink raw milk and consume raw cheese if available.
2. Hemp milk and coconut milk are good alternatives as well as organic almond and rice milk in moderation.
3. Consume cultured organic milk products in moderation. Organic Pastures is a California based milk company that sells good quality milk. Drink only whole milk.
4. Consume processed milk products very sparingly, if at all. This includes processed cheeses and yogurt. Purchase hormone free milk and milk products, as well as Greek yogurt.
5. Remember, calcium is derived from other food sources such as: lamb, amaranth, broccoli, kale, greens and sardines, seeds, and nuts.

Wine

Wine was commonly used in Biblical times for blessings, medicinal purposes, and for joyous occasions. The Greeks' wine was made from water and grapes. Sometimes the Greeks sweetened their wine with honey or made medicinal wine by adding thyme, pennyroyal and other herbs. The wine today, however, is not the same as wine back then. The wine was much more diluted in comparison.

There were also stern warnings about overconsumption and the intemperate use of strong drink in biblical references. Very wise advise and applicable for today. Even though it was a living food created by God for our consumption, if we abuse what God has given us, there will be consequences. Although society generally deems drinking alcohol as socially acceptable, it is often used to numb pain, numb stress, or used as an artificial relief from emotions. Alcoholism is one devastating consequence of abuse of alcoholic drinks. Alcohol is addictive, high in unnecessary calories and is nothing more than fermented sugar. Once in the body it is converted to glucose (blood sugar). If one has a sugar addiction and goes off of sugar, be aware that alcohol does not become a substitute. Other effects of intemperance that scripture warns about are the redness of the eye in Genesis 49:12, improper speech in Proverbs 20:1 and Isaiah 28:7, and distorted judgment in Proverbs 31:5.

> *And Noah began to be a farmer, and he planted a vineyard. Then*
> *he drank of the wine, and was drunk, and he became uncovered*
> *in his tent.*
>
> Genesis 9:20-21

Here we see above with the story of Noah, the consequences of too much wine. There are many references in scripture about the use of wine for various intents as noted in the scriptures below. The verses no not condone intoxication, rather indicates that wine was used for medicinal purposes in ancient times.

> *Then Melchizedek king of Salem brought out bread and wine: he*
> *was the priest of God Most High.*
>
> Genesis 14:18

> *And you shall bring as the drink offering half a hin of wine as an*
> *offering made by fire, a sweet aroma to the Lord.*
>
> Numbers 15:10

> *….And wine that makes glad the heart of man….*
>
> Psalms 104:15a
>
> *Give strong drink to him who is perishing, and wine to those*
> *who are bitter of heart. Let him drink and forget his poverty and*

remember his misery no more.

Proverbs 31:6-7

Go eat your bread with joy, and drink your wine with a merry heart; for God has already accepted your works.

Ecclesiastes 9:7

No longer drink only water, but use a little wine for your stomach's sake and your frequent infirmities.

1 Timothy 5:23

Another consequence to our health is that alcohol can deplete the brain of chemicals and overwhelm the liver with toxins. The free radicals produced by alcoholic drinks can inflame the liver leading to scar tissue. Cirrhosis of the liver is one consequence. When this happens toxins can't be filtered out and nutrients can't get in. Some signs of weak liver function (not necessarily due to alcohol consumption only) might include any of the following: burping after eating, pain or tightness in the right shoulder area, potbelly, sensation of fullness just under the right rib cage, cravings for fried foods, hot feet at night, yellowness in whites of eyes, varicose veins or spider veins, skin problems, brown spots on backs of hands, red dots on skin, edema, bruising easily, or bloating after eating.

Wine was part of offerings, blessings, used for celebrations, as well as for healing. But Paul in Ephesians issues a stern warning for over consumption of wine.

And do not be drunk with wine, in which is dissipation; but be filled with the Spirit.

Ephesians 5:18

Benefits of wine

Researchers at UC-Davis have found that wine contains a group of chemicals in red wine called saponins (strong antioxidant-also found in olive oil and soy beans). This has been shown to help reduce cholesterol.

Another chemical called resveratrol has been shown to help reduce the risk of heart disease. Red wines contain 3-10 times more of these chemicals than white wines. The highest amounts are found in: Red Zinfandel, then Sirah, then Pinot Noir and Cabernet Sauvignon.

Wine also effectively kills bacteria. This effect is not necessarily due to the alcohol content but rather the polyphenols in the wine. Polyphenols are antioxidants that have the ability to scavenge free radicals. Even though there are benefits, you can get the resveratrol in other products.

A recent study in the British Medical Journal reported that a study designed to evaluate wine for any antimicrobial effects found that it was by far the most powerful of the 3 mixtures studied (wine-bismuth salicylate-ethanol).[21] This study explains why wine has been used as a digestive aid since biblical times.

Again, alcohol is nothing more than fermented sugar and can be very addictive. Use wine in moderation and avoid the use of other alcoholic beverages.

What about Coffee?

Oh, yes, the best part of waking up! First of all, coffee did not exist in biblical times. The origins date back to the 9th century in Ethiopia and entered America in the 16th century.[58]

Second, coffee is a narcotic beverage. It contains caffeine. For most of our existence, our pattern of sleeping and wakefulness depended on the sun and the seasons. In biblical times, caffeine was not needed. People depended on the sun and their healthy adrenals to wake themselves up. With the advent of the industrialized revolution and schedules built around the sun with indoor jobs timed by a clock, humans had to learn to adapt. Caffeine became therapeutic as a wake promoting substance.

Not only is it considered a drug, it is an addictive substance. Caffeine stimulates the adrenal glands to release an adrenaline-like substance. According to Kathy Freston, "Caffeine stimulates the central nervous system by tricking the brain (*deception again!*), into ordering the release of excess adrenaline. This excess adrenaline in the body builds up in the muscles, creating body tension, headaches, and muscle spasms. And because the adrenal glands are being artificially stimulated by a chemical, they may not have ample time to rest and rejuvenate themselves and may become depleted and weak. This in turn, results in increased feelings of exhaustion, even when the brain is ordering the release of adrenaline. One may find themself needing more and more caffeine to feel awake or even normal."[13]

People typically rely on caffeine to cover up a sense of depletion. Eating high quality fats like butter, coconut oil, or eggs will help restore the balance of energy metabolism. It also causes alterations in your calcium to phosphorous balance and over stimulates your glandular system. Combined with the stomach hydrochloric acid it forms a potent toxin called caffeine hydrochloride. As this toxin absorbs into your portal circulation and hits your liver, bile is released in attempt to flush it from your system. This is one possible explanation for people who have better bowel regularity by drinking coffee.

Third, coffee is acid producing. Holding a cup of coffee lowers one's bodily frequency 8MHz and taking one sip can lower it 14MHz. It can take up to three days for the body to recover from one drink of coffee. So, is 8 or 14 MHz good news or bad news? Living things survive on MHz values. The higher the MHz, the higher the frequency, the healthier your body, and the more "alive" is the plant. Rose Essential Oil has a MHz value of about 350; the highest of the plant's Essential Oils. Canned foods have a value of less than 32. Lowering your body's MHz 8-14 values significantly impairs the body's frequency.[49] Low frequencies lower the acid environment and breed disease. Disease cannot survive in a more alkaline or highly oxygenated state.

Coffee also depletes the system of Thiamin, a B vitamin, and leads to fatigue, nervousness, general malaise, aches and pains. It is a diuretic which then leads to dehydration. It also can deplete the adrenal glands. Since caffeine is a nervous system stimulant it causes the adrenals to secrete adrenaline, the hormone that your body depends on during emergencies to elevate your heart rate, increase respiration and blood pressure for a rapid fight-or flight response.[47] When coffee is over-used, the adrenals can become exhausted. If a person depends on coffee to keep going, then they have developed a caffeine sensitivity and have exhausted their adrenals.

Besides B vitamins, regular use of coffee inhibits minerals from being properly absorbed in the small intestine. Coffee causes unnecessary excretion of calcium, magnesium, potassium, iron, and trace minerals into the urine. All these minerals are necessary for good health and prevention of osteoporosis. Also, Coffee breaks down into a by-product known as uric acid. This acid is known to burden the kidneys, contributing to kidney stones and gout.

Next, caffeine forces the liver to release glycogen into the blood stream. The pancreas responds to the sudden increase in blood sugar by releasing insulin. Insulin is a hormone that can cause excess carbohydrates to be stored as fat. Within an hour or so later, the body has a sharp decrease in blood sugar. This creates a hypoglycemic, or low blood sugar state, and now the body senses a desire to have another cup of coffee to keep going.[50] This sets up a viscous cycle.

Lastly, de-caffeinated coffee is no better than regular coffee. Both contain toxins called **trichloroethylene,** which is a de-greasing agent in the metal industry and solvent in the dry cleaning industry, as well as **pesticides like dieldrin, chlordane, and heptachlor, chlorogenic acid, nitrosomine, and caffeine.** Other toxins that are associated with coffee consumption include the following:

- Tap water which is loaded with **pollutants**
- Grounds were ground months or years ago sitting **oxidizing** in an **aluminum** can
- Opened cans initiate further oxidation process
- Grounds poured into **bleached** filters
- Brewing **oxidized** fats on top of **pesticide, chlorinated, aluminum, and bleached (dioxin)** toxins
- Reheated coffee releases 400% more **caffenol** into the body
- Poured into a **styrofoam (styrene)** cup

- Add to that **Aspartame**-which breaks down into **formaldehyde**
- Add to that milk laden with **hormones and antibiotics**

And what do we do every Sunday? Bring that cup of coffee into church while we listen to the Sunday sermon and afterwards ask for prayer for healing because we have fatty liver, aches and pains, kidney stones, insomnia, acid indigestion, gallstones, osteoporosis, ulcers, anxiety, and other symptoms associated with coffee use.[37]

So, is there anything good about coffee? Well, antioxidants have been found in coffee. According to Caroline Leaf, PhD, "Coffee beans are extraordinary complex fruits that contain over 1000 phytochemicals. It also has the power to help prevent most major killers including cardiovascular disease, cancer, diabetes, liver disease and Alzheimer's disease." Leaf continues to say that "a number of case-controlled human studies, compared to coffee abstainers, showed that those who drank pure black organic coffee cut their risks of breast cancer by 57% and diabetes by 67%." "Research has even shown coffee to help reduce DNA damage, which in turn inhibits cancer and aging. Scientists are beginning to discover that coffee's phytochemistry exerts direct biological actions on the body, weaving a complex web of indirect protective effects, one of which is neuroprotective (helps prevent diseases of the brain and cognitive decline)." "Coffee also reduces inflammatory activity and improves metabolism. However, there is a lot missing from commercial coffee beans so one has to be careful of what you drink," reminds Leaf.[23] Due to the fact that this is a hot beverage, it increases body temperature. However, considering all the toxins (there have been documented over 1,000) that went into making that cup of Java, I seriously doubt that the amount of antioxidants left in that cup are doing your body any good. It still is not the best or primary source of antioxidants. There are plenty of antioxidants in fruits and vegetables, which Americans are sorely lacking.

The small benefits simply do not out-weigh the risks. We are a nation addicted to caffeine. The extent of our society to coffee addiction is clearly obvious with the lines of cars waiting for coffee orders at drive-through coffee shops. Sitting with a cup of coffee in hand listening to the Sunday sermon is a far cry from the people sitting at the feet of Jesus at the Sermon on the Mount. There was no coffee around then to keep them awake. But is one cup once in a while bad? No, moderate amounts are healthy especially if it is organic, freshly ground, filtered with an unbleached filter and served in a ceramic or paper mug. Enjoy that cup! [50]

What about tea?

Although I could not personally find any reference to tea in   scripture, tea has been around since 2737 BC. It was originally consumed as a medicinal drink in China. There are many varieties and benefits of drinking tea. First, immune boosting compounds. Tea is rich in polyphenols like catechins and flavonoids which function as antioxidants.

Second, tea can aid in digestion and calm nerves.

Third, alertness from the caffeine can also improve mood and memory. It has also been shown to reduce the risk of heart disease by acting on LDL cholesterol and triglycerides.

One caution I wish to point out is that tea can contain fluoride and too much drinking of tea might affect your bones and result in skeletal fluorosis. Black and Green tea have the highest content and has the potential of harming bones but also interfere with thyroid function.

What about Soda and Energy Drinks?

Soda and Energy drinks did not exist in ancient times. Recently Coca-Cola has set itself the goal of raising consumption of its products in the United States by at least 25 percent a year, and because the adult market is stagnant, selling more soda to kids has become one of the easiest ways to meet sales projections, says Eric Schlosser.[43] Sodas contain sugar and caffeine. Twenty years ago, teenage boys in the United States drank twice as much milk as soda; now they drink twice as much soda as milk.

Energy drinks are the worst invention of the 21st century next to cell phones. Their popularity is exclusive to the United States and have been popular since 1977 with the debut of Red Bull. France banned Red Bull after an 18 year old athlete died from drinking four cans. Since Red Bull's debut, more than 500 drinks have been launched in the last 30 years. This amount to 5.7 billion dollars in profits for the industry.[25] These drinks were manufactured for a generation that recently has become sleep deprived, energy deprived, and addicted to sugar. Previous generations before the invention of soda or energy drinks have not depended upon canned drinks for their baseline energy.

Why are energy drinks so detrimental to the body? They contain massive amounts of sugar: some up to 102 grams. This creates a demand for insulin on your body to combat the excess. Sugar increases inflammation. And many sodas and energy drinks use the worst kind of sugar: High Fructose Corn Syrup. They also contain stimulants such as caffeine (as much as 80-150 mg. per serving), ginseng, and taurine that give the consumer jolts of energy and high amounts of carbohydrates. Even though these are stimulants, they have been known to cause insomnia, high blood pressure, rapid heartbeat, difficulty breathing, seizures, anxiety, and heart palpitations. The sugary taste and the boost of energy can be very addictive.[63] Because the drinks contain caffeine, they are diuretics and cause loss of fluids. If a person isn't getting the recommended water intake and substitutes fluids with Monster or Red Bull, or others, they are at high risk of dehydration. Fatigue is one sign the body does not have enough water intake.

With up to 30g of sugar, the fallout of this is that it will cause energy levels to crash once the sugar leaves the bloodstream. This sugar rush is short lived, so the consumer is soon feeling more fatigued than they were to begin with. To stay energized another drink is consumed to stay awake or alert and the cycle of addiction continues until one day they crash and can't figure out why this happened.

Caffeine is the main ingredient that gives energy.[25] However, the amount of caffeine is three times that as one cup of coffee. Caffeine can lead to diseases such as osteoporosis, insomnia, and ulcers. Guarana is one ingredient that contains caffeine. One gram of guarana equals 40 mg of caffeine, and may increase the total caffeine in the drink.[18] Some side effects noted in studies include nervousness, irritability, sleeplessness, increased urination, abnormal heart rhythms, decreased bone levels, and stomach upset.[18]

Other ingredients found in soda and some energy drinks are aspartame- a neurotoxin, and phosphoric acid- an antagonist to calcium leading to osteoporosis, bone loss and dental caries.

Our bodies were created, by God's design, to produce energy from cellular respiration, foods, water and air. The adrenals are responsible for the "fight" or "flight" reactions to stress. The energy drinks, due to the stimulants, cause a response from the adrenals. If the body is already under a great amount of stress from work load, homework, relationships, etc., which already tax a person's adrenals, and another stressor of energy drinks is added, that is abusing the temple of God and the consequence is adrenal burnout. Adrenals are needed for blood sugar regulation, metabolism, sex hormone regulation, and brain function—to name a few. So, besides adrenal burnout, the body is placed at risk of a domino effect with other organs or systems failing.

Although marketing campaigns claim benefits to improve endurance, enhance immune system, improve memory, promote excretion of toxins, weight loss, decrease triglycerides, suppress appetites, lower risk of diabetes (What? With 30g of sugar per serving, how can that possibly lower risk of diabetes?), and improve sexual performance, the scientific evidence does not exist to support most of these claims.[18] And, the benefits just simply do not out-weigh the health risks nor do they justify the continued use of energy drink products. Remember, marketing is for the industry's profits, not our health. Deception again.

Our bodies were not created to handle such high doses of these ingredients. At some point we will eventually suffer the consequences. I know personally of one teenager who over-consumed some energy drinks to stay awake for final exams and ended up hospitalized for serious dehydration. The doctors told her she was lucky to still be alive. Instead of going to bed at a reasonable time that our bodies require, by God's design, consumers are sabotaging their sleep, and then end up becoming dependent on a stimulant to keep their bodies awake.

In comparison, people in ancient civilizations never needed "energy" from drinks. They relied on their healthy functioning adrenals, pure clean water, and adequate sleep cycles to keep their bodies going. What does this say about our state of health that we can no longer depend on our adrenals and brain function to keep us awake? This is truly sad. Good pure water with citrus juice is a great alternative, and our brains and adrenals will function far better on this drink.

But this is what I commanded them, saying, 'Obey My voice, and I will be your God, and you shall be My people. And walk in all the ways that I have commanded you, that it may be well with you.''

Jeremiah 7:23

10

. . . . . .

Our Emotions and Stress

Beloved, I pray that you may prosper in all things and be in health, just as your soul prospers.

3 John 1:2

These early apostles cared about the health of their fellow Christians. So ought we through prayer and hospitality.

Or do you not know that your body is the temple of the Holy Spirit who is in you, whom you have from God, and you are not your own? For you were bought at a price; therefore glorify God in your body and in your spirit, which are God's.

1 Corinthians 6:19-21

Knowing that our bodies are the temple of the living God should say something about its value, how we treat it, and should be a warning to us if we abuse it, misuse it, ignore it, and treat it wrongly.[47] This reference to God in 1 Corinthians 6 above is attaching the importance of actions reflecting our belief about our body being a temple. It is a reference to holiness of the entire community; that some things build up and some things destroy it. Our actions and lifestyles must reflect this belief because, again, we are not our own. We were intended to serve others. We must use the body as it was intended. Charles Stanley says that the "kind of wisdom that promotes good health involves God's viewpoint of the human body."[47]

In the Old Testament the tabernacle was an actual tent where God's spirit dwelled. In Exodus 40:34-38 we see that the temple was honored and treated with respect because of God's presence there. Since our bodies are temples where the spirit of God lives, should we treat them with less honor and respect than a physical building?

What we eat, drink, how much and how well we sleep, and how much stress we encounter, and how we handle emotions all plays a part in our health. It's hard to focus on serving others when our body is crying out for help. The Bible does not condemn the display of emotions or feelings. In fact, burying feelings can lead to hardness of heart and apathy. The immune and digestive system are also impacted by negative thoughts and emotions. Therefore, keeping our thoughts in captivity is a ruling handed down by God because He knows what will happen to our bodies on a physiological level.

God created us with the capacity to express a variety of emotions, yet holding onto unhealthy emotions for long periods of time has dire consequences on our overall health. We see warnings of this also in scripture. God has given us guidelines to renew our minds so that we can have hope in healing.

Throughout life we all face situations that evoke emotions. How we handle them needs to honor God. The results of our handling will affect our health; for better or for worse. It is important to confess our feelings as well as to identify the sources. We may not like the idea of digging around our soul to pull out the root of our emotions, but if emotions are not dealt with, then we could spend our life treating symptoms with drugs, while the "hidden cancer," as Charles Stanley refers, of resentment spreads and takes over our life. Serious emotions, such as bitterness and resentment require radical care, not a bandage or flippant dismissal.

Ephesians 4:26 warns us to not let the sun go down on our wrath. We are to deal with emotions and not let them take root. It has been alleged that the root cause of most illness is stored emotions. Thoughts always precede emotions and we have the ability to change our thoughts. Anger, resentment, unforgiveness, and a desire for revenge all trigger the classic alarm triad response to stress – adrenal gland hypertrophy (enlargement or swelling), thymus and lymph gland atrophy (shrinkage) and gastric inflammation. This state can potentially rob us of our health and shorten our lives.

Thoughts influence every decision, words, action, and physical reaction we make.[21] Caroline Leaf, Ph.D. states that every time you have a thought, it is actively changing your brain and your body — for better or for worse.[23] She continues to present two choices: we can let our thoughts become toxic and poisonous, or we can detox our negative thoughts, which will improve our emotional wholeness and even recover our physical health.[23] Consider while undergoing a health treatment program to partake in an emotional release program. By learning to control our thought life and experience emotional release, we will be able to lead an emotionally sound and physically healthy life.[23]

Stress

Stress has many causes, but is closely related to emotions. Dr. Leaf contends that stress is the direct result of toxic thinking and that stress is harmful when it is sparked by negative emotions.[23]

> *Have mercy upon me, O Lord, for I am in trouble; my eye wastes away with grief, Yes, my soul and my body! For my life is spent with grief, and my years with sighing; my strength fails because of my iniquity, and my bones waste away.*
>
> Psalm 31:9-10

Here in Psalm 31 David was crying out about his grief and distress. His strength was failing due to the stresses of life. And again, in Psalm 51 below, his spirit was overwhelmed.

> *Have mercy upon me, O God, according to your lovingkindness; according to the multitude of your tender mercies, blot out my transgressions. Wash me thoroughly from my iniquity, and cleanse*

me from my sin. For I acknowledge my transgressions, and my sin is ever before me. Against You, You only, have I sinned, and done this evil in your sight— that you may be found just when you speak, And blameless when you judge. ....Purge me with hyssop, and I shall be clean; wash me, and I shall be whiter than snow. Make me to hear joy and gladness, that the bones which you have broken may rejoice. Hide your face from my sins, and blot out all my iniquities. Create in me a clean heart, O God, and renew a steadfast spirit within me.

Psalm 51:1-10

Therefore I say to you, do not worry about your life, what you will eat or what you will drink; nor about your body, what you will put on. Is not life more than food and the body more than clothing?

Matthew 6:25

.....Casting all your care upon Him, for He cares for you.

1Peter 5:7

Two thousand years ago Jesus commanded us to not worry as recorded in Matthew above. This rebuke is in our best interest because He knew that stress could lead to physical problems and we are now learning in the medical field why stress is so detrimental to our health. In the passage above, Jesus offers a simple solution on how to respond to worry: pray. Remember that God is our refuge for whatever emotions we experience.

Stress is defined as the outward circumstances over which you have **no** control or circumstances or influences over which you **do** have control, inward attitudes, beliefs and thought patterns, or internal physical conditions. Since stress begins with perception, our thought life can have a significant effect on our physical health. These physical conditions can include an acidic environment from acid foods, junk food, thermal stress, and stressful lifestyles. Stress produces high acid levels in our body by draining it of acid-reducing minerals such as calcium and magnesium.

Stress also causes our cells to increase in activity producing more acidic waste. Over time our body could potentially become exhausted from this cycle and possibly lose its ability to defend itself against sickness and disease.

How does the stress response work? First, we perceive a threat; physical, emotional, cognitive, spiritual, behavioral, or relational. Then physiologically we enter in full alert. Our limbic system kicks in and releases chemicals into the body. These chemicals produce many hormones such as adrenaline, which makes nutrients available to the body for strenuous action, noradrenaline, which increases blood pressure and blood flow to the muscles to enable us to move, as well as cortisol and DHEA, and glucocorticoids, which makes fat available for energy and increases alertness in the brain.

Next, our pupils dilate to give us clearer vision; our breathing increases, giving our body more oxygen to burn the added fuel, and now we can act with more strength and speed. We either fight or flee the threat or stressor. Cortisol becomes available to calm down the body. Over time with this constant state of stress response, without time to recover, the accumulated effects wreak havoc on the body and causes numerous states of degenerative health affecting the digestive system, skin, heart and circulatory system, blood sugar, fertility, neurotransmitters, and immune system to name a few. In order for us to maintain health, the adrenal hormones need to be in balance, and we need to maintain proper pH balance through the healthy foods outlined above.

Handling Stress

How can we handle stress?

» First through prayer and meditation.

Pray without ceasing.

1 Thessalonians 5:17

The writers of both Old and New Testament knew the necessity of resting in the Lord with prayer. Prayer affects us and acknowledges our dependence on God's grace and power in every aspect of life, and helps us to focus on seeking first His kingdom and righteousness. It is at His feet that we can find rest in His mercy and draw strength from His promises of help in times of stress or need. In biblical times possible stressors were war, famine, or wild beasts. In comparison, some of our current stressors are jobs, relations, economy, or terrorist's plots.

» Eat foods containing nutrients that support the adrenals and aid in lowering Cortisol. Foods that contain Vitamin B, A, D, E, K along with foods high in Amino Acids such as Taurine (fish/animal protein, Vitamin B6, Cysteine), Tyrosine (wheat germ, cottage cheese, asparagus, spinach, lentils), and Glutamine (dates, oranges, apples)

» Take Adaptogenic herbs such as: Ginseng, Echinacea, Ashwaghanda root, Reishi, etc.

» Special supplements as directed from a nutritionist or health care practitioner may need to be taken if the adrenals are severely stressed._

» Daily times of deep relaxation should be performed 1-2 times per day for 5-10 minutes

» Get adequate sleep to avoid sleep deprivation. Research published in Lancet demonstrated that chronic sleep loss produces serious health risks mimicking the effects of aging and early diabetes. Avoid staying up too late. Research has shown that 1 hour of sleep before midnight is equivalent to four hours afterward.

» Listen to calming music.

» Take a vacation. (Europeans take 8-10 weeks per year. Americans struggle with 2-3 weeks).[18]

Caution: Watching T.V. may not be restful. By definition, watching television is a recreational activity. Halting breathing and nail biting during intense drama episodes is not relaxing.

11

. . . . . .

Is Exercise Biblical?

Exercise

In ancient times people did not need gyms for exercise. Exercise was their life. Running, riding horses, swimming, walking, rowing, constructing fortresses and canals, cooking, washing clothes, planting and gathering food are examples of what was common physical activity in the ancient life. The Olympics began in Olympia in 776 B.C. but were possibly held many years prior to that time. The games consisted of foot races, long jump, wrestling, spear throwing, boxing, and chariot races. Races were also held in Delphi, Corinth, Caesarea, and Athens. Isthmian games were held every two years in Corinth. Winning was the prime importance and usually the winners were awarded crowns of olive or palm branches, honors, gifts, and special privileges. The athletes were said to have trained for 10 months. The games continued every four years until A.D. 394 when Emperor Theodosius of Rome abolished the games as part of a series of reforms against pagan practices.[20]

Several examples in the scripture references below relay the message that physical exercise was practiced, but not in the same context as we know it today. Now we have become a society of sedentary lifestyles that have prompted the surge of gym clubs with promises of restoring health.

Your rowers have brought you out into the high seas. The east wind has wrecked you in the heart of the seas.

Ezekiel 27:26 (RSV)

And he will spread out his hands in the midst of it as a swimmer spreads his hands out to swim; but the Lord will lay low his pride together with the skill of his hands.

Isaiah 25:11 (RSV)

For bodily exercise profits a little, but godliness is profitable for all things, having promise of the life that now is, and of that which is to come.

1 Timothy 4:8

Ezekiel and Isaiah are two examples that confirm physical activity was a way of life. Timothy here is referring that physical exercise is good for us, but that godliness is preferable. We can exercise all we want for whatever purpose, but that it is useless if we do not have a relationship with Christ.

Our bodies were created to move. Lymph does not move on its own. It needs bodily movement or massage to move and do its job of removing waste. Joints need lubricating and movement helps to lubricate those joints. Muscles will atrophy if not moved. Exercise improves blood flow and oxygen levels, refreshes our body, renews our energy, oxygenates us, and strengthens our muscles and stamina. Other benefits include regulating blood pressure, reducing inflammation, improving mood and concentration. If our bodies are stagnant they become a breeding ground for disease and disorder Stagnant or sedentary lifestyle has been linked to one-third of cancer. deaths. Even simple movements and exercise decreases the risk of certain diseases. On the other hand, we should not be using physical exercise as the answer to inner contentment.

People of ancient times were active in manual labor from sun up to sun down. They mostly walked, or ran, wherever they needed to go, or rode on camel or horses. Jesus himself was a carpenter which means his occupation was manual labor. His livelihood took him thousands of miles of walking. Women were not sedentary. They took care of household chores. The laundry alone was a days' work.

According to a recent ABC news special, currently the world's longest-lived people in Costa Rica don't pump iron, run marathons, or join gyms. They move their bodies without thinking about it. They walk to places instead of driving. They climb stairs. They garden in their yards.

Countless studies show that sedentary lifestyles contribute to disease.

According to Carol Ruvolo, physical and spiritual fitness are actually built up and strengthened by the rigorous activity of strenuous exercise. While diet and rest support that activity with energizing nourishment and rejuvenating refreshment, skipping meals when we're busy, or eating poorly, steals the energy we need to keep going, and lack of rest saps our strength for the work of the day. Important fluids and nutrients are lost when exercising, so it is critical while undertaking an exercise routine to replenish the body's water and mineral status and to incorporate more antioxidant rich foods such as greens, berries, and citrus. Good nutrition and rest are essential if we are to exercise well.

12

· · · · · ·

Remedies of the Bible

When Jesus saw him lying there, and knew that he had already been a long time [in that condition], He said to him, "Do you wish to get well?"

John 5:6 (NAS)

And Isaiah said, Take a lump of figs. And they took and laid [it] on the boil, and he recovered.

2 Kings 20:7 (KJV)

The passage in Kings is evidence that God's people knew about the plants that God provided and used them liberally to help with healing. Figs are high in vitamins A, C, K, calcium, magnesium, potassium, and fiber. They contain phytosterols (which are cholesterol lowering properties), as well as antioxidants and anti-inflammatory properties commonly used for boils. High water content is also contained in figs.

Physicians of old used a variety of remedies to help the sick return to health. Common practices included fermentations, baths, fasting, soups, juices, enemas, suppositories, ventilation, purges, essential oils, music, mudpack and compresses. A liquid broth of honey and water, or barley gruel was also common.[20] Food and plants of the earth were the medicine of that time period.

When he had said these things, He spat on the ground, and made clay with the saliva; and He anointed the eyes of the blind man with the clay. And He said to him, "Go, wash in the pool of Siloam," (which is translated, Sent.) So he went and washed, and came back seeing.

John 9:6-7

It is here that we see the first recording of mud packing by Jesus. One commentator stated that Christ cured many who were blind by disease or accident; here he cured one born blind. Thus he showed his power to help in the most desperate cases, and the work of his grace upon the souls of sinners, which gives sight to those blind by nature. He continues to expound that human reason cannot judge of the Lord's methods; he uses means and instruments that men despise.[56]

Numerous research studies show the use of mud in health therapies since the time of Hippocrates. Throughout its history, the benefits of therapeutic mud baths have been recognized as preventative and curative. Peat and mineral mud baths have been used in central Europe for the last 200 years for treating arthritis and other disorders. Now, according to Robert Marshall, PhD, of Premier Research Labs, the use of mud packs have shown to have many beneficial health effects such as increasing circulation, boosting immune system, easing muscle tension, rejuvenation of cells, restoring nerve and energy flow, increased mineralization, and clearing whole body toxic bioaccumulation.[26]

And so it was, whenever the spirit from God was upon Saul, that David would take a harp and play it with his hand. Then Saul would become refreshed and well, and the distressing spirit would depart from him.

1 Samuel 16:23

Music as therapy began thousands of years ago. The above scripture is one illustration of an account where music was used to restore a person's emotional health. In this case it was King Saul who was delivered through the use of music with David's harp.

The Bible mentions 128 plants and herbs used in everyday life in the ancient near-east, at least 33 species of essential oils, and more than 1,000 references to their use in maintaining wellness, acquiring healing, enhancing spiritual worship, purification from sin, and setting apart individuals for holy purposes. They were the medicines of ancient civilizations.

Health care, or "sick care" as it is referred to today, is not what it used to be. When people were sick in biblical times, they did not run to Kaiser or their local pharmacy to get a drug for all their ailments. They used the plants, the herbs of the field and essential oils, provided by God, as common remedies for ailments. The healers and physicians of biblical times were the priests and teachers.

Allopathic health care today consists of medical doctors, nurses, midwives, diagnostic labs, pathology clinics, and health facilities with various specialties. These specialties consist of optometry, occupational therapy, gastroenterology, endocrinology, dermatology, allergy, orthopedic, cardiology, pediatrics, pharmaceuticals, and the rest who provide preventive, curative, rehabilitative, or palliative care to individuals and families. The care is typically based on treating symptoms. This systematic way of care did not exist until the 1880's.

It wasn't until 1901, the beginning of the industrialized revolution, that organized medicine took hold. According to Robert Marshall, PhD, 5% of income was spent on health care in 1901. At that time only 5% of the U.S. population was chronically ill. By 1929 the first medical insurance company, Blue Cross, was created as a way to help hospitals' revenue and to keep care at reasonable costs. In stark contrast, 16% of income was spent on health care in 2010, but the percentage of chronically ill Americans was 50%. Dr. Marshall attributes this to the food we are eating and how it is grown and the conventional remedies Americans are using.[26]

Another alternative to conventional medical practice that has been around since the early 1800's is homeopathy. According to the National Center for Homeopathy, homeopathy is a system of medical therapy that uses very small doses of medicines, or remedies, that are prepared from any substance found in nature including plants, animals, and minerals. Homeopathy is based on the Law of Similars. This Law of Similars has its history as far back as Hippocrates in 400 B.C., but didn't come to light until the early 1800's with Dr. Samuel Hahnemann, a German medical doctor. The Law of Similars means that "like cures like." These remedies are in minute, or micro, doses and are used to stimulate the body's innate healing powers. What makes homeopathy so unique is the preparation process. According to Lenia Scanlon of *Natural and Synthetic Medication*, the microdoses are prepared by taking an extract of the original substance and putting it through a series of dilutions. Between each dilution, the preparation is succussed, or vigorously agitated with impact which is believed to capture the living essence or biological information of the herb, mineral, or plant. With every step of dilution and succussion, the potency or strength of the substance is increased making it more effective as a therapeutic modality. Homeopathics are generally regarded by the FDA as safe due to this extreme dilution.

As a "rare jewel in the mainstream of medicine" some of the benefits of homeopathy include:

- Alleviating symptoms
- Releasing toxins from storage sites in tissues
- Facilitating drainage of toxins and their elimination from the body
- Desensitizing the body of allergic reactions
- Neutralizing the action of free radicals

Could it be that if we used methods that worked two thousand years ago, two hundred years ago, or with more natural methods, that we might see a difference in the skyrocketing health statistics?

Essential Oils-What Are They?

Essential oils, other "rare jewels in the mainstream of medicine," are the plants' life force and carry electrical charges measured in MHz value of 52-320. Processed food has a value of less than 32 Hz! [49] This equates to little if any life force. Essential oils are the plants' immune system warding off undesirable viruses and bacteria. Essential oils regulate plant growth and can serve many of the same purposes for us as they do in plants.[49] In contrast to pharmaceuticals, there are no negative side effects, they do not lie to cells, and are non-toxic. Just as the bleeding resins of plants fill the wound and initiate the healing process for the plant, pouring of essential oils into cuts and wounds can accelerate healing and protect from infections because of their antiseptic and oxygenating capabilities. These oils are composed of very small molecules able to pass through all tissues of the plant and cell walls, through the blood-brain barrier and the skin. For example, one drop of peppermint oil on the bottom of the foot can be tasted in six seconds.[49] Essential oils have the highest ORAC (oxygen radical absorbance capacity) value of any substance in the world. For example, one ounce of clove oil has the antioxidant capacity of 120 pounds of blueberries.[49] Antibiotics have serious side effects and contribute to bacterial overgrowth and stronger dosages needed over time. Essential Oils are a healthy alternative. When essential oils are used to attack bacteria, they are selective because they are imbued with God's intelligence. They know which are the bad guys and which are the good ones so that when they have killed off the bacteria causing the sickness, the good bacteria are still alive to serve us.[49]

Essential Oils are inhaled, taken internally (only those approved by the FDA for consumption), or applied topically by rubbing or massaged. The Hebrew and Greek word for "anoint" means to rub, cover, or smear with oil. A commonly used Hebrew word for anoint was "masach"-similar to our English word "massage." It is also the root of the term "Messiah." The Greek term "Kristos" "Christ" means "anointed one."[49]

Most of the references to oils in scripture were to olive oil, but many oils were used for a variety of purposes and are referenced numerous times in The Bible. Though not an exhaustive list, below are a few of these references. Frankincense and myrrh are commonly known as two oils presented to the Christ child. Oils were used as cosmetics, fuel for lamps, healing agents, meal offerings, and articles of commerce. Ointments, which were prepared from oils were used also for anointing, cosmetics, burials, and used on the skin and hair. More references can be found in the back of this book in the Reference section.

Exodus 12:13, 22-23 –**Hyssop** - *And the blood shall be to you for a token upon the houses where ye [are]: and when I see the blood, I will pass over you, and the plague shall not be upon you to destroy [you], when I smite the land of Egypt. And ye shall take a bunch of hyssop, and dip [it] in the blood that [is] in the bason, and strike the lintel and the two side posts with the blood that [is] in the bason; and none of you shall go out at the door of his house until the morning. For the Lord will pass through to smite the Egyptians; and when he seeth the blood upon the lintel, and on the two side posts, the Lord will pass over the door, and will not suffer the destroyer to come in unto your houses to smite [you].*

The hyssop plant was used in the Old Testament when the doors of the houses were painted with blood to protect them. The Essential Oil of hyssop has commonly been used as an anti-inflammatory, and protectant against bacteria, and infections. The berries of the hyssop plant are called capers.

Exodus 29:7-**anointing**- *Then you shall take the anointing oil, and pour it on his head and anoint him.* (NAS)

Leviticus 8:30-**anointing**- *So Moses took some of the anointing oil and some of the blood which was on the altar, and sprinkled it on Aaron, on his garments, on his sons, and on the garments of his sons with him; and he consecrated Aaron, his garments, and his sons, and the garments of his sons with him.* (NAS)

Leviticus 14:15-18-**anointing**- *The priest shall also take some of the log of oil, and pour [it] into his left palm; the priest shall then dip his right-hand finger into the oil that is in his left palm, and with his finger sprinkle some of the oil seven times before the LORD. And of the remaining oil which is in his palm, the priest shall put some on the right ear lobe of the one to be cleansed, and on the thumb of his right hand, and on the big toe of his right foot, on the blood of the guilt offering; while the rest of the oil that is in the priest's palm, he shall put on the head of the one to be cleansed. So the priest* *shall make atonement on his behalf before the LORD.* (NAS)

Numbers 11:7- **Coriander**-*Now the manna was like coriander seed, and its appearance like that of bdellium.*

Exodus 16:31 *And the house of Israel named it manna, and it was like **coriander** seed, white; and its taste was like wafers with honey.*

Psalm 23:5-**anointing**- *You prepare a table before me in the presence of my enemies; You anoint my head with oil; My cup runs over.*

Psalm133:2-**precious**- *It is like the precious oil upon the head, Coming down upon the beard, [Even] Aaron's beard, coming down upon the edge of his robes.* (NAS)

Isaiah 41:19-Essential Oil **plants** were present- *I will put the cedar in the wilderness, the acacia, and the myrtle, and the olive tree; I will place the juniper in the desert, together with the box tree and the cypress.* (NAS)

Ezekiel 27:19—**accessible** in markets- *Vedan and Javan traded with yarn for thy wares: bright iron, cassia, and calamus, were among thy merchandise.* (ASV)

Mark 6:13-**anointing and healing** purposes for those who were sick- *And they were casting out many demons and were anointing with oil many sick people and healing them.* (NAS)

Luke 10:34b-**healing** oil- *and went to him and bound up his wounds, pouring on oil and wine; then he set him on his own beast and brought him to an inn, and took care of him.* (RSV)

James 5:14-15-**anointing and healing**- *Is any among you sick? Let him call for the elders of the church, and let them pray over him, anointing him with oil in the name of the Lord; and the prayer of faith will save the sick man, and the Lord will raise him up; and if he has committed sins, he will be forgiven.* (RSV)

What about Supplements?

The earth brought forth vegetation, plants yielding seed according to their own kinds, and trees bearing fruit in which is their seed, each according to its kind. And God saw that it was good.

Genesis 1:12 (RSV)

God originally made the land to produce vegetation that would supply us. Supplements were neither invented nor necessary in ancient times. The people had the herbs of the field and the essential oils as their "supplements." Over time and through sin, selfishness, and poor farming practices in the last 100 years, the land has been stripped of nutrients that it once held. Vitamin and minerals are catalysts to speed up necessary chemical reactions in the body yet supplements should never be a substitute for eating healthy.

> *But in the seventh year there shall be a sabbath of solemn rest for the land, a sabbath to the Lord. You shall neither sow your field nor prune your vineyard.*
>
> Leviticus 25:4

We see here in Leviticus that the people were instructed to rest the land for a time. Although for a spiritual purpose, the principal is applicable. Crops need to be rotated to yield quality mineral content.

Since our food is grown on progressively mineral deficient soil with over one billion pounds of pesticides, synthetic fertilizers, and other pollutants used per year, and now increasing in Genetically Modified or Genetically Engineered, our food is nutrient deficient and toxic laden, escalating the need for supplementation.

> *You shall not sow your vineyard with different kinds of seed, lest the yield of the seed which you have sown and the fruit of your vineyard be defiled.*
>
> Deuteronomy 22:9

Again the above scripture is speaking spiritually, however, a lesson can be garnered from the wisdom. Besides the lack of crop rotation, many farmers use hybridized seeds. God warned of the consequences of this in the book of Deuteronomy. These fruits and vegetables from hybridized seeds cannot reproduce their own kind which causes a decrease in the nutrition available to us. According to the USDA in 1994, the average

American diet is significantly lacking in the essential minerals needed for energy production and protection from free radical damage.

As Robert Marshall, PhD, states, "In order for the immune system to handle this challenge, taking quality nutritional products to supplement our diets is not a luxury anymore, but a necessity for those in search of lasting health."[26]

Not all vitamins are created equal and we see deception in the supplement industry as well as the pharmaceutical industry. It is a common principle now to eat foods from plants and not foods made in a plant. This same principle can be applied to supplements. Supplements made in a laboratory by a chemist are synthetic, unless the packaging states, "whole or live, or once living"food source. These synthetic forms may contain toxic tag-alongs, or excipients, such as sugars (disguised by names such as maltodextrin or sucralose), herbicides, pesticides, fumigants, artificial colorings, artificial flavors, fillers and preservatives such as magnesium stearate, silicon dioxide, methylcellulose, propylene glycol, parabens, sodium benzoate, and others.[26] The fillers are used to hold the ingredients together or to keep the ingredients from sticking to equipment during the mixing process. These fillers and excipients also allow the manufacturing process to be faster and easier which keeps the cost of the product lower.

Take magnesium stearate. This chalk-like substance has lubricating properties which prevents the pills from sticking to each other and allows the machinery to run faster and smoother. According to Dr. Mercola and his research, stearic acid suppresses T cells which are the natural killer cells in the body and an important component of our immune system. Stearic acid, according to studies, causes the collapse of cell membrane integrity. Over time this can destroy cellular functioning.

Take ascorbic acid. This is a synthetic vitamin C and derived from cornstarch, corn sugar, and volatile acids mixed in a fermentation process.[12] Very detrimental for someone who has a corn allergy.

According to Fitzgerald, synthetic vitamin E comes from an Eastman Kodak plant where it is a by-product of an emulsification process used to manufacture film. After the purification process it is sold to supplement companies.[12]

Even though to a chemist synthetic and natural vitamins may look similar, they don't assimilate the same way in the human body. Synthetics and excipients in supplements eventually lead to adverse health effects including inflammation and increase the toxic load in a person's body.

Supplements made from whole foods or once living sources resonate with the body. Believing that our bodies don't know the difference between synthetic and natural, we have indoctrinated ourselves into believing that just taking any vitamin supplements will keep us healthy. The body knows, by God's design, what is foreign and what is real, and what creates life force and what creates inflammation. When choosing supplements keep in mind those that maintain ideal cellular resonance (whole food based), are excipient free, and are packaged in dark or opaque containers to block light. Be wary of purchasing supplements on the internet or from companies that appeal to your emotions. Purchase from your health care practitioner, naturopathic practitioner, or a certified nutritionist who can guide you into choosing supplements that are right for your body and your health needs.

The following are some of the important supplements necessary and the food sources available:

Antioxidants - These are free-radical scavengers that prevent oxidative stress on the body. They are abundant in blueberries, greens, green tea, and foods with vitamin C. While a relatively new word in modern times, God knew we needed these foods from the beginning of time. These foods were not known for their properties until recently, but have sustained people for thousands of years.

Vitamin A - Helps to manufacture protein and DNA. Available in carrots, pumpkins, yams, fish, beet greens spinach, and eggs.

B Vitamins - These are lost in the refining and cooking process. Drinking tea, coffee, and alcohol further diminishes our supply. Vegetarians often lack B_{12}. B vitamins help with the nervous system, muscles, brain function, cell processes, energy production and amino acid metabolism, vision, red blood cell formation. These vitamins come from meats, vegetables, eggs, fish, and milk. It is best for maximum absorption to use whole live source B vitamins.

Vitamin C - Essential in wound healing and facilitates recovery from burns and illness, helps form healthy teeth, gums and bone, essential to protein collagen formation, vital for immune function, supports iron absorption, and strengthens blood vessel walls. This is abundant in citrus fruits and the Camu Camu plant.

Vitamin D - Essential to help increase intestinal absorption of calcium, maintains proper blood levels of phosphorus and calcium, necessary for strong bones and bone function, strengthens immune system. Our sun is still the best source.

Enzymes - To help digest proteins, carbohydrates, and fats. Enzymes are responsible for using the vitamins and minerals as building materials for our body functions. Organic fruit and vegetables, milk, and honey in their raw form contain live enzymes.

Omega 3 fatty acids- These are the core building blocks of our cell membranes and affects all cellular functions and communications. Essential fats provide energy and insulation, nourishes and strengthens cell membranes, and controls inflammation. Fish, nuts, and flaxseed oil are still valuable sources.

Supplements- Who Needs Them?

- Those with:
- Busy lifestyles
- Compromised immune systems
- Food allergies
- Non-organic food intake
- Pregnancy
- Smokers
- Calorie restricted diet
- Strict vegan diets
- Those over fifty years old, due to loss of vitamins and malabsorption difficulties

SUMMARY

Food Isn't What It Used to Be: Biblical Principles for Today

Pray and spend time with devotions and meditating on scripture. In the Hebrew mind if disease were to be healed, the first step was to restore the relationship with the Lord. Evaluate our relationship with our Creator in regard to this subject of health. Pray for our food and be thankful to God for where and how the food came to the table.

Commit to discipline thoughts, temptations, what we put in our mouth, and what comes out of our mouth. As long as we are living in this world, we can be continually seduced or tempted by what could lead us into ill-health. Dr. Brian Clement once said that it is difficult for most of us to remain self-disciplined about what we put in our bodies and on our bodies in the face of so many cultural temptations to remain lazy or gluttonous.[12] He continues to impart that our internal saboteur often triumphs because most of us are slaves to our food habits and our cravings for the conveniences of modern life, and that the more intense our cravings for harmful foods, the greater the likelihood we also will develop biochemical deficiencies and imbalances.[12] Let it not be so with us. Practice what the author in Hebrews, Philippians, and 1 Corinthians below exhorts and lay aside the weights of temptations and to not give up:

Therefore we also, since we are surrounded by so great a cloud off witnesses, let us lay aside every weight, and the sin which so easily ensnares us, and let us run with endurance the race that is set before us.

Hebrews 12:1

Not that I have already obtained this or am already perfect; but I press on to make it my own, because Christ Jesus has made me his own. Brethren, I do not consider that I have made it my own; but one thing I do, forgetting what lies behind and straining forward to what lies ahead, I press on toward the goal for the prize of the upward call of God in Christ Jesus.

Philippians 3:12-14 (RSV)

No temptation has overtaken you that is not common to man. God is faithful, and he will not let you be tempted beyond your strength, but with the temptation will also provide the way of escape, that you may be able to endure it.

1 Corinthians 10:13 (RSV)

Carefully choose your food and drink, and what you purchase.

- Shop at your local farmer's market, food co-op or CSA.
- Look for the USDA Organic label on foods. This is a legitimate claim to being certified organic. It's one of the few programs run by the USDA that actually has integrity.
- Read the ingredients labels! If you see names of chemicals you can't pronounce, don't buy it.
- Buy more unprocessed food ingredients and make your own meals rather than purchasing ready-to-eat, processed foods, which are almost universally formulated with disease-promoting ingredients.
- Grow some of your own food! The best food you can ever eat, and trust, is food from your own garden. Share your bounty with friends.

Avoid the following:

Acrylamides - Toxic, cancer-causing chemicals formed in foods when carbohydrates are exposed to high heat (baking, frying, grilling). Also called Advanced Glycated End Products. They are present in everything from bread crusts to snack chips, charcoaled meats, and because they aren't intentional ingredients, acrylamides do NOT have to be listed on labels.

Additives- Additives are chemicals used to preserve, color, flavor, and market the food products. Think about the bright colors on foods marketed for kids-candy, cereals, snacks, etc. Kids love bright colors. These bright colors are fully laden with chemicals that mostly come from coal-tar petroleum and can cause a multitude of allergic reactions, brain reactions, and behavioral functions. Some hidden additives are: MSG, BHT, BHA, propyl gallate, sodium nitrite, sodium nitrate, sodium benzoate, sulfur dioxide, benzoic acid, and sodium bisulfate, aspartame, magnesium stearate, Blue #1, 2, Red #3, Yellow #6, Green #3, High Fructose Corn Syrup.

Artificial Flavoring- The name tells you it is fake!

Aspartame - A neurotoxin and prevalent in diet sodas and chewing gum.

Autolyzed Proteins – Highly processed form of protein containing free glutamate and used to mimic the taste-enhancer chemical MSG.

BPA (Bisphenol-A) – A hormone mimicking chemical found in nearly all food packaging plastics including water bottles, prepared food, and packaged produce. Active in just parts per billion, BPA promotes cancer, infertility and hormone disorders. It also "feminizes"males, promoting male breast growth and hormone disruption.

Canned fruits in syrup- These are devoid of nutrients and are high in sugars.

Canned vegetables—These are devoid of nutrients. Choose fresh or frozen as much as possible.

Casein – Milk proteins.

Corn Syrup

Food Colors – FD&C Red #40, for example, is linked to behavioral disorders in children. Nearly all artificial food colors are derived from petroleum, and many are contaminated with aluminum. These are in any packaged food stuff from gummy vitamins, medications, to toothpaste. Read labels carefully.

Fortified foods- These are usually a form of processed foods. This is done by stripping away the nutrients in a food and then putting the nutrients back in the food synthetically.

Fragrance – When the word "fragrance"is listed on a label, it means a synthetic fragrance made in a test tube from any of over 200 synthetic chemicals. They are very cheap, toxic imitations of real herbal scents. These "fragrance"chemicals, which can accumulate in your organs, can cause many symptoms, such as headaches, lung problems, skin irritation, dizziness, memory impairment, rash, and more.[26]

Genetically Modified Ingredients – Not currently listed on many of the labels because the GMO industry (Monsanto and DuPont) absolutely does not want people to know which foods contain

GMOs. Laws are changing however. Nearly all conventionally grown corn, soy, certain brands of oatmeal, and cotton are GMOs. They're linked to severe infertility problems and may even cause the bacteria in your body to produce and release a pesticide in your own gut. If you're not eating organic corn, you're most certainly eating GMO corn.

High Fructose Corn Syrup

Hydrochloride - When you see anything hydrochloride, such as Pyridoxine Hydrochloride or Thiamin Hydrochloride, those are chemical forms of B vitamins that companies add to their products to be able to claim higher RDA values of vitamins. But these are synthetic, chemical forms of vitamins, not real vitamins from foods or plants. Nutritionally, they are near useless and may actually be harmful for you.

Hydrolyzed Vegetable Protein – A highly processed form of (usually) soy protein that's processed to bring out the free glutamate (MSG). Used as a taste enhancer.

Over using Medications- All medications have side effects and can destroy the intestinal lining and normal bacteria of the gut as well as throw off normal functioning of physiology. Drugs do not "cure"illness. Use wisely.

Parabens – These are preservatives used to inhibit microbial growth in skin, hair, and other products including many supplements. They are highly toxic and can cause allergic reactions and skin reactions.[26] These have also been implicated in raising estrogen levels leading to estrogen dominance: a leading cause in breast cancer.

Partially Hydrogenated Oils - Oils that are modified using a chemical catalyst to make them stable at room temperature. This creates trans fatty acids and greatly increases the risk of blocked arteries. It also promotes what is called "sludge blood,"which is thick, viscous blood that's hard to pump. This is usually diagnosed by doctors as "high blood pressure"and treated with blood-thinning medications.

Phosphoric Acid – The acid used in sodas to dissolve the carbon dioxide and add to the overall fizzy-ness of soda. Phosphoric acid will eat steel nails. It destroys tooth enamel. Search Google Images for "Mountain Dew Mouth"to see photos of teeth rotted out by phosphoric acid.

Propylene Glycol – A synthetic petrochemical liquid used in the automotive industry to winterize RVs and emulsify creams and lotions, and in the medical industry in the colonoscopy prep solutions. It can be absorbed through your skin and potentially cause allergic reactions. It's also used to make the fake blueberries you see in blueberry muffins, bagels and breads, and is in most beauty products.

Sodium (Table Salt) - The processed white salt lacking in trace minerals. In the holistic nutrition industry, we call it "death salt"because it promotes disease and death. Real salt, on the other hand, such as sea salt or pink Himalayan salt, is loaded with the trace minerals that prevent disease, such as selenium (cancer), chromium (diabetes) and zinc (infectious disease). Much like with bread and sugar, white salt is terrible for your health. And don't be fooled by claims of "sea salt"in grocery stores. All salt came from the sea if you go far back enough in geologic time, so they can slap the "sea salt"claim on ANY salt! Purchase from only reliable sources.

Sodium Lauryl Sulfate - This is a caustic detergent used because it is cheap and sudses well. It is used as an engine degreaser and garage floor cleaner. Research shows that SLS has a degenerative effect on the cell membranes and denatures protein such as in hair or skin. SLS can corrode hair follicles and inhibit hair growth contributing to hair loss.[26] This is a common ingredient in hair care products.

Sodium Nitrite – A cancer-causing red coloring chemical added to bacon, hot dogs, sausage, beef jerky, ham, lunch meats, pepperoni and nearly all processed meats. It is strongly linked to brain tumors, pancreatic cancers and colon cancers. The USDA once tried to ban it from the food supply but was out-maneuvered by the meat industry, which now dominates USDA regulations. Sodium nitrite is a complete poison used to make meats look fresh. Countless children die of cancer each year from sodium nitrite-induced cancers.

Soy Protein – This is the number one protein source used in "protein bars,"including many energy bars widely consumed by bodybuilders. Soy protein is the "junk protein"of the food industry. It's usually made from genetically modified soybeans (often grown in China) and then subjected to hexane, a chemical solvent that can literally explode.

Sucralose - Splenda; a chemical.

Sugar – Remember moderation is the key here.

Textured Vegetable Protein - Usually made of soy protein which is extracted from genetically modified soybeans and then processed using hexane, an explosive chemical solvent (see Soy Protein, above). Widely used in vegetarian foods such as "veggie burgers" (most of which also contain MSG or Yeast Extract).

Yeast Extract - Hidden form of MSG that contains free glutamate and is used in many "natural" food products to claim "No MSG!" Yeast extract contains up to 14% free glutamate. You'll find it in thousands of grocery store products, from soups to snack chips. I even once spotted it used on fresh meat!

Keep hydrated with water daily.

Detox/cleanse/fast at least once or twice per year.

Exercise regularly at lease 2X a week as well as play: play with your children; your pets.

Watch portion sizes.

Consume heart healthy fats instead of heart clogging fats.

Get adequate sleep and go to bed at reasonable times.

Daily relaxation and stress reduction

Enjoy adequate sunshine, without sunscreen for your skin type, regularly along with vitamin D supplement.

Use super foods, herbs, homeopathic immune boosters, and essential oils to promote health.

Make a plan for parties and outings with friends. These events put dietary temptations into your path. Food is central in our society for social comfort and breaks the ice for conversations. Browse through the food table to find what you can eat and stick with the plan. Or, eat a small meal before you leave then you won't be as hungry and tempted to load up on anything to fill your hungry desires. With children, give them choices. Provide healthy substitutes.

Birthday parties: If you give the message that when we're

celebrating, we're having a good time and it's all right to eat the fun non-nutritious foods we don't ordinarily eat, then you are setting up a judgment that the day-to-day more nutritious foods are dull and boring. This is the wrong message and will hinder the progress of you and your family and make it harder for healthy foods to become a way of life. If you must have a birthday cake, then try healthier alternatives like adding carrots, zucchini, and nuts to the recipe.

Focus on the memorable games, entertainment, and decorations. Food is only a part of the party and can be healthy and delicious as well for these occasions.

Try having a theme of brunch or lunch and serve food as a cafeteria style where children can make their own sandwiches and or salads. Have a yogurt bar with bowls of dried fruits, nuts, maple syrup, and yogurt so guests can make their own yogurt sundae.

Plan your meals. The old phrase, "If you fail to plan, then you plan to fail" applies. Planning meals really does help and by now your family can help with the planning. Menus can be designed and posted in the kitchen. One idea is to have a one day a week that is "child's choice." Your child would plan all the meals for that day and even help with the shopping and preparation. Or, you might have a "child's breakfast" weekend where your child plans the breakfasts for the weekend (keeping in mind the biblical pantry).

Pay attention to deception in food ads. We have an enemy who seeks to deceive and distract us from becoming all that we can be. Prepare for this with discernment and discretion. Take heed that little compromises can destroy our health.

Afterword

Remember, it is much more difficult to regain health when we lose it than to keep it while we are healthy. Clearly the thrust of these biblical principles is to prevent ill health before it arises. From a biblical health perspective, many diseases can be prevented by taking wise precautions.

Whether it is junk food, gluttony, dietary indiscretions, lifestyle indiscretion choices, the Devil's deceptive antics, not eating enough, uncontrolled emotions, over exercising, under exercising, or any other "weight," or hindrance, we are bearing, let us lay aside those things that prevent us from being all that God has called us to be.

Lastly, food is to nourish, not nurture. Be ready to present your bodies as a living and holy sacrifice, acceptable to God, which is your spiritual service of worship, as stated in Romans 12:1. George W. Calver, a medical doctor for the U S Congress in 1928 stated, "Give 5 percent of your time to keeping well. You won't have to give 100 percent getting over being sick."

I hope that you have gained some knowledge in how food has changed over time and that what we eat, how we manage our stress, what we choose to help our infirmities does matter with our overall health. It is evident that we do not need current research to support this. Our forefathers knew this and recorded it for our knowledge throughout The Bible. Arthur Pink states, "The scriptures speak for themselves."[31] It is my prayer that your health will be restored, allowing you to continue your walk in the path God has put before you. (3 John 1:2) As the blind man in John 9:6 obeyed Jesus and took the steps of faith that brought healing, so too may you obey the Lord with steps of faith so that you may be healed.

— Christine Andrew, CNC

APPENDIX

Essential Biblically-Based Whole Food Pantry

Herbs & Spices	Whole Grains & Legumes	Protein
Basil	Amaranth	Eggs
Cinnamon	Oats	Goat cheese,
Chicory	Spelt	aged, raw cheese
Coriander	Millet	Meat-lamb, chicken,
Cumin	Teff	venison, beef
Dill	Quinoa	Yoghurt, Kefir
Garlic	Wild Rice	Butter
Ginger	Lentils	Fish -Salmon, halibut,
Milk Thistle	Barley	sardines, cod, sole,
Mint	Corn	herring
Sage	Dried beans-kidney,	
Aloe	black, chickpeas, navy	
Rosemary	Wheat (Sprouted, whole grain-Ezekiel Bread)	
Turmeric		
Sea Salt		
Fennel		
Hyssop/Capers		
Dandelion leaves		

Nuts & Seeds

Almonds
Cashews
Pecans
Walnuts
Sunflower seeds
Sesame seeds
Flaxseeds

Oils & Condiments

Honey
Olive Oil
Grape seed Oil
Flaxseed oil
Butter
Vinegar
Sunflower Oil
Capers
Vegetable stock
Walnut oil

Beverages

Milk (whole, raw)
Goat's milk
Wine (moderation!)
Water

Dried Fruit

Cranberries
Apricots
Raisins
Figs
Dates

Produce

Seasonal Fruit and vegetables
Onions, leeks
Greens
Apples, grapes, pears,
Berries
Figs
Citrus (lemons, oranges, grapefruit)
Pomegranates
Cucumber
Sea vegetables (kelp)
Olives
Melons

SNACK IDEAS

Flaxseed crackers-(Crunchmaster brand)
Cheese slices with seasonal fruit slices, or vegetable slices

Seasonal vegetable slices with or without dip
Olives
Hardboiled egg, egg salad
Yogurt-plain Greek yogurt with fruit added
Nuts

Sample Ancient Meal Plan

	Roman (ientaculum)	Greek (akratismos)
Breakfast:	Porridge (Creamy Rice Cereal) Honey, salt Eggs Cheese Olives Water	Barley bread dipped in wine Figs, olives Pancakes
	(prandium)	(ariston)
Lunch:	Bread Fruit Salad greens Eggs Meat/fish Cheese Vegetables	Light meal of: Meat Soup (Vegetable)
	(cena)	(aristodeipnon)
Dinner:	Eggs, oysters, lettuce Wine with honey	Olives

~ ~ ~ ~   ~ ~ ~ ~

Bread

Bread (Wheat or barley)

Onions

mixed with cheese or honey

Vegetable

Vegetables- cabbage, onions,

Eggs

lentils, sweet peas, beans boiled

Soup- Legumes, milk, cheese

or mashed, seasoned with

Meat- lamb, fish kabobs

olive oil, Vinegar and herbs

Fruit- apples, figs, dates, grapes,

Meats- Fowl, fish, cattle, rabbit

pears, cheese, honey

Cheese, garlic, onion

Wine

~ ~ ~ ~

Fruit- figs, raisins, pomegranate

Wine

Chestnuts

Eggs- soft or hard boiled

Curdled milk

Dinner: Barley Bread
Lentil Stew
Cucumber yogurt Salad
Date Walnut Bread

RECIPES

Broccoli Quinoa
Recipe from Carmen Anderson

   3 cups cooked quinoa
   5 cups raw broccoli, (or other seasonal vegetable) cut into small
      florets and stems
   3 medium garlic cloves
   2/3 cup sliced or slivered almonds, toasted
   1/3 cup freshly grated Parmesan cheese
   2 pinches Himalayan salt
   2 tablespoons fresh lemon juice
   1/4 cup olive oil
   1/4 cup heavy cream
   Optional toppings: basil, chili oil (see under Miscellaneous for
   homemade recipe), sliced avocado, feta or goat cheese

Pre-cook quinoa according to directions and drain any extra water. Heat the quinoa and set aside.

Now, barely cook the broccoli by pouring 3/4 cup water into a large pot and bringing it to a simmer. Add a pinch of salt and stir in the broccoli. Cover and cook for a minute, just long enough to take the raw edge off. Transfer the broccoli to a strainer and run under cold water until it stops cooking. Set aside.

To make the broccoli pesto, puree two cups of the cooked broccoli, the garlic, 1/2 cup of the almonds, parmesan, salt, and lemon juice in a food processor/blender. Drizzle in the olive oil and cream and pulse until smooth.

Just before serving, toss the quinoa and remaining broccoli florets with about 1/2 of the broccoli pesto. Taste and adjust if needed. You might want to add more of the pesto, salt or lemon juice a bit at a time. Turn out onto a serving platter and top with the remaining almonds, a drizzle of the chili oil, and some sliced avocado or other optional toppings.

Serves 4-6

Brussels Sprouts Shaved with Bacon, Leeks, and Pomegranate Seeds
From Lynda Abeyta

2 pounds of Brussels Sprouts
5 slices bacon, chopped
1 leek, sliced
1 clove garlic, minced
2/3 cup chicken broth
¼ teaspoon sea salt
Pinch of black pepper
2-4 tablespoons of pomegranate seeds

Shred the Brussels Sprouts using a food processor until slightly coarse.

Cook the bacon in a large skillet or stockpot set over a medium-high heat until crisp.

Remove the bacon from the pan, and set aside, leaving the grease in the pan.

Add the Brussels sprouts, leeks, and garlic to the pan and saute for 5 minutes.

Add the chicken broth, sea salt, and pepper. Cover and steam for 5 minutes, until the sprouts are bright green and tender. Return the bacon to the pan.

Garnish with pomegranate seeds and serve warm.

Serves 6

Cake Made with Oil
From Israel

2 cups semolina flour
4 cups cold water
½ teaspoon salt
1 cup olive oil
¼ teaspoon dried sage
Honey

Toast the semolina in a large ungreased pan, stirring constantly, for about 2-3 minutes. Place it in a bowl, and add the cold water and salt. Mix well.

Return mixture to pan and cook over a medium flame, stirring constantly, until the mixture thickens to the texture of a slightly dry porridge, about 7 minutes.

Remove from the flame and allow to cool. Slowly pour in the olive oil, and continue mixing until it is well absorbed.
Wet hands and form handfuls of the dough into round, plump cakes about the size of large cookies. Place on an ungreased pan and bake for 10-15 minutes in a medium oven.

Drizzle about ½ teaspoon of honey on each cake after removing from the oven and before it completely cools.

Carrots with Cumin
Miriam Feinberg Vamosh-Biblical Recipes

6 medium carrots
Water
Sea salt
1 tablespoon raw honey
½ teaspoon ground cumin
Black pepper
¼ cup olive oil
2 cloves garlic, minced
1 tablespoon parsley, chopped

Peel and slice carrots into ¼-inch slices. Put in a pot with a little water and salt. Cook covered for about 10 minutes until tender but still crisp.

Mix remaining ingredients and add to the hot carrots. Toss and adjust seasoning to taste.

Serve as a side dish with roasted lamb.

Cucumbers and Onions with Rue and Mustard Dressing
From Cooking with the Bible

6 large cucumbers
3 large sweet onions
2 teaspoons ground mustard
¼ teaspoon cumin
½ teaspoon rue*
¼ cup pine nuts
2 teaspoon honey
½ cup cider vinegar
3 garlic cloves

Use rue sparingly in this cucumber and onion salad; parsley may be substituted if desired.

Peel the cucumbers and slice into long strips.

Place in a steel bowl. Chop the onions into small pieces and add them to the cucumbers.

In a small food processor, grind the mustard, cumin, rue, and pine nuts. Place them into a mixing cup and add honey and vinegar.

Peel and press 3 garlic cloves into the mixture. Pour over the cucumbers and onions; cover. Refrigerate for at least 1 hour, and serve cold.

Yield: 6–8 servings

*Rue has been known to have an adverse effect on some diners; parsley can be substituted if one wishes, although the results are a bit different in taste.

Cucumber and Yogurt Salad

3 large cucumbers, peeled and sliced thin
Juice of one lemon
1 clove garlic, minced
4–5 sprigs fresh mint, finely chopped
1 pint yogurt (plain whole milk Greek Yogurt)
½ teaspoon salt
Salad greens mix

Lay cucumbers in a chilled glass bowl. Squeeze the juice of one lemon over the cucumbers. Sprinkle half the minced garlic and finely chopped mint leaves over the salad greens. Toss the other half of the mint and garlic into the yogurt, then add the salt. Pour the yogurt mixture over cucumbers and refrigerate one hour before serving. Serve the cucumber and yogurt as the dressing over the salad greens.

Fennel and Sun-dried Tomato Stuffing

2 loaves sourdough bread, or a whole grain bread, cut into 1-inch pieces
1 stick butter
4 fennel bulbs, trimmed and coarsely chopped, fronds set aside
3 cups chicken broth
1 cup sun-dried tomatoes (packed in oil), chopped
2 tablespoons balsamic vinegar
1 teaspoon dried oregano
Salt and pepper

Preheat oven to 300 degrees. Spread the bread pieces on a baking sheet.

Bake 35 to 40 minutes until lightly toasted.

Melt 6 tablespoons of butter in a large saucepan over low heat. Add the fennel and increase heat to medium. Cook, stirring until tender.

In a medium pot over medium heat, add the chicken broth and the sun-dried tomatoes. Simmer for 10 minutes.

In a large baking dish, toss together the toasted bread, fennel, tomato-broth mixture, balsamic vinegar and oregano. Add salt and pepper as desired.

Cover dish and bake for 20 minutes. Melt remaining 2 tablespoons of butter, uncover dish and brush stuffing with the butter. Bake uncovered until the bread browns, about 10 minutes.

Garnish with fennel fronds.

Greek Salad

Grape tomatoes sliced in half (Tomatoes did not appear until 15th century, but this salad tastes better with the tomatoes)
Slices of sweet onion
Diced peeled cucumber
A handful of olives
Top with Feta Cheese

Dress with finest quality extra virgin olive oil and vinegar dressing or Pomegranate Dressing

Serve with whole grain bread.

Grilled Fish

½-1 cleaned, whole fish per person (Tilapia, Trout, Cod)
Olive oil
Salt and pepper
Sumac
Sprig of thyme, hyssop or oregano (or ½ teaspoon each of dried herbs)
Grape leaves, if available

Brush the outside of each fish with olive oil.

Sprinkle the fish inside and out with salt, pepper, and sumac.

Place a sprig of thyme, and a sprig of hyssop or oregano inside the fish.

If grape leaves are available, wrap each fish in them before putting it directly on the grill.

Cook for about 8 minutes on each side or until done.

Honey Cake
From Israel

6 eggs
¼ teaspoon cinnamon
1 cup sugar
¼ teaspoon instant coffee
$^1/_3$ cup olive oil (or avocado oil)
$^1/_8$ teaspoon ground cloves
7 ounces water
½ honey
3 cups flour
1 tablespoon baking powder

Whip eggs with the sugar. Slowly add and continue to whip into the egg mixture the oil, water and honey. When mixed well, add the flour, baking powder, cinnamon, coffee and cloves.

Pour into a greased and floured 9"x13" pan and bake 350⁰ for about 30 minutes until inserted wooden pick comes out clean.

Laban Immu
From Gems in Israel
Source: Oded Schwartz

This delicious recipe comes from Lebanon. It is an example of an ancient Middle Eastern classic and it could be the dish that is indicated in Genesis 18:1-8.

Yoghurt or soured milk was one of the staples of nomadic life. Researchers go even further and maintain that consuming soured milk protected our forefathers against bovine tuberculosis. Soured milk also acts as a meat tenderizer and is used extensively both in Middle Eastern and Indian food as a marinade for grilled or roasted meats.

Ingredients:
1 kg boneless shoulder or leg of veal or young lamb, cubed into 2.5 cm cubes
10 small onions
4-5 sprigs of fresh thyme
500 ml. yoghurt
Juice of 2 lemons
1 tablespoons flour or cornstarch
1 egg, well beaten
3 tablespoons butter or Samna
2 tablespoons dry mint or 4 tablespoons fresh chopped mint
2 cloves of garlic, mashed

Preparation:
Place the meat in a heavy pan and, just cover with water. Bring to a boil, skim and simmer for 30 minutes. Add the onions and the herbs and go on simmering until the meat is tender. Adding a little water if it gets too dry.

Beat the cornstarch and egg into the yoghurt and transfer the mixture into a small pan. Stir constantly over medium heat until just boiling. Pour over the meat and mix well. Simmer for a further 5 minutes or until the sauce has thickened.

Heat the butter in a small frying pan. Add the mint and garlic and sauté gently for 3-4 minutes or until the garlic has started to change color.

In a large heated serving bowl arrange the meat and some of the sauce over a mound of bulgur and pour the hot sautéed mix on top. Decorate with mint and serve.

Serves: 6

Lamb Stew
Christine Andrew. CNC

1 pound of lamb (shoulder or breast meat)
2 tablespoon olive oil or avocado oil
2 cups of chicken stock
2 tablespoons tomato paste
2 cups new potatoes
6 carrots
3 white turnips
1 cup peas
1 cup green beans
 small onions

Cut lamb into pieces. Brown meat in skillet in the oil. Remove to a Dutch oven.

Pour off fat from skillet. Put in 2 cups of stock and 2 tablespoons tomato paste. Bring this to a boil in the skillet. Pour over meat. Simmer, covered.

Peel and cut potatoes, carrots, turnips, onions. After lamb has cooked 1 hour, skim off fat, add vegetables to the pot and simmer covered for 1 hour longer.

Add peas and beans, fold in. Sprinkle with parsley.

Lebanese Mint, Egg, and Onion Omelet
From Cooking with the Bible

6 eggs
½ cup light cream
1 tablespoon flour
A dash or two of paprika
Salt and pepper to taste
1 cup olive oil
½ each red, green, and yellow peppers, finely chopped
1 medium onion, finely chopped
½ teaspoon sumac
4 sprigs fresh mint (leaves only), chopped

Preheat oven to 350°F.

Crack the eggs into a bowl and beat them by hand until light in color. Slowly stir in the cream, flour, paprika, salt, and pepper; set aside. Heat a large skillet and fry the peppers, onion, and sumac in olive oil until the ingredients are soft and somewhat mushy. Line a small but deep ovenproof pan with the peppers and onion mixture, and pour the egg combination over it. With a sharp knife on a hard cutting board, gather the mint leaves together and cut them finely, then chop them into small pieces. Mash with a mortar and pestle or in a small bowl using the handle end of a table knife. Stir half of the mint into the omelet fixings; sprinkle the rest on top. Cook for 15–20 minutes or until the surface is just beginning to brown.

Yield: 4 servings

Meat Loaf
Christine Andrew, CNC

1 small onion, chopped
1 tablespoon olive oil
½ pound lean ground beef (grass-fed beef)
½ pound ground dark meat turkey
2 tablespoons flaxseed meal
1 small can tomato paste
½ cup water
½ tablespoon Nutritional Yeast (Premier Research Labs)
1 egg yolk, lightly beaten
1 tablespoon chopped parsley
1 teaspoon ground dried red chilies
Salt and pepper to taste

Preheat oven to 350 degrees. Sauté onion in oil until golden. Combine remaining ingredients and mix well. Bake in a greased loaf pan for about an hour until browned.

Rhonda's Minestrone Soup
From Rhonda Malkmus of Hallelujah Acres

8 cups Simple Vegetable Soup Stock
14 ounce can organic unsalted Italian tomatoes
15 ounce can organic garbanzo beans
15 ounce can organic red kidney beans
1 cup carrots cut into small thin chunks
1 cup finely shredded cabbage
1 cup celery, cut into ¼ inch lengths
1 cup onion, diced
½ cup fresh parsley, minced
2 cloves garlic, minced
½ teaspoon dried oregano
½ teaspoon dried basil
½ teaspoon thyme
1 teaspoon Sea Salt
1 package spiral noodles, prepared according to directions

Directions:

Drain and rinse kidney and garbanzo beans, or soak dried overnight.

Sauté garlic, parsley, carrots, onion, celery, cabbage in a small amount of soup stock until onions are translucent.

In a large soup pot, place soup stock, tomatoes and all remaining ingredients. Simmer until cabbage is tender.

Place some noodles in individual soup bowls and ladle soup over the noodles and serve.

Red Lentil Soup
From Israel

1 pound of red lentils, washed
1 tablespoon olive oil
½ cup chopped coriander
5 garlic cloves, chopped
Juice of 2 lemons
1 teaspoon sea salt
½ cup flour
1 cup cold water

Cook lentils in about 2½-3 quarts water until soft.

Heat oil in skillet and fry chopped coriander and garlic.

Add juice of lemons and salt.

Mix and add to soup ½ cup flour and 1 cup cold water.

Add coriander, garlic, and lemon mixture to soup. Let simmer for about 10-15 minutes.

For heartier soup, add 1 chopped onion and ½ pound of chopped and cooked bacon.

Serves 6-8

Winter Romaine Salad
From Israel

1 head of romaine lettuce
1 red onion
½ cup walnut halves
2 cups mandarin orange slices

Dressing:

½ cup avocado oil
¼ cup rice vinegar
½ teaspoon salt
½ teaspoon paprika
½ teaspoon white onion, grated (or onion powder with parsley)
½ teaspoon Mustard Seed Aromatic Seasoning (Israel Za'atar)
½ teaspoon celery seed

Directions:

Tear lettuce into bite sized pieces and place in a bowl.

Slice onions into thin rings. Slice in quarters and add on top of the lettuce.

Peel and separate mandarins into slices and add to the lettuce.

Sprinkle the walnuts on top.

Mix dressing ingredients together. Add dressing to salad just before serving.

Whole-grain Pancakes
Christine Andrew, CNC

1 cup buckwheat flour

½ cup Brown Rice flour

½ cup Almond meal

2 teaspoons double-acting baking powder

1 teaspoon baking soda

1 teaspoon Premier Pink Salt

2 beaten eggs

¼ cup melted butter

2 cups buttermilk, or whole milk with a teaspoon of vinegar

1 teaspoon vanilla

Mix dry ingredients in a bowl. Mix wet ingredients in a separate bowl. Add wet ingredients to dry ingredients. Fold until blended. Cook on a greased hot griddle. Serve with fresh whipped cream, cheese, honey, or fresh fruit.

Makes about 16 pancakes

Polish Jewish Beet Soup

From Tony Gruska, chef/owner Monticello Restaurant of Davis, California- A Seasonal Cuisine restaurant

4 to 5 large beets
Juice of 1 to 2 lemons
1 to 2 potatoes, quartered
1 onion, chopped
1 cup chicken stock
2 tablespoons sugar
2 tablespoons fresh dill, chopped

Scrub beets, Cover with water and boil with juice of 1 to 2 lemons until soft, about 40 minutes. Remove from the water. Let cool slightly, peel and dice. Return diced beets to water. Add onion and potatoes. Stir in chicken stock and sugar. Adjust the sweet and sour to your own taste with sugar and lemon. Sprinkle chopped dill over soup when ready to serve.

Pomegranate Dressing
From Christine Andrew, CNC

¼ cup fresh lime juice

¼ cup pure Pomegranate juice- (Pomegranate Elixir from Premier Research Labs)

1 tablespoon sour cream or Vegenaise

1 teaspoon Dijon mustard

1 teaspoon Stevia

¼ teaspoon ground cumin

1 garlic clove, minced

4 tablespoons Olive oil

Salt

Combine first 7 ingredients in a bowl. Add olive oil and whisk to blend. Season with salt to taste.

Potato Salad (Potatoes came about in the 15th Century)
From Christine Andrew, CNC

1 pound (3 large) potatoes, cooked and cut into small chunks
1 red pepper, chopped fine
1-2 tablespoons green onions chopped fine
1 carrot, chopped fine
1 small can black olives, chopped fine
2 stalks celery
2-4 tablespoons yogurt or Vegenaise
1 teaspoon prepared mustard
½ teaspoon of garlic
1 teaspoon dried thyme
Pepper to taste

Combine mayonnaise and seasonings. Add to vegetables and potatoes. Toss gently and refrigerate until chilled.

Pumpkin Flax Muffins

2 ¼ cup flour

1 cup pureed pumpkin

½ cup Flaxseed meal

¾ cup Sour cream

¾ cup Honey or Turbinado sugar

1/3 cup Milk

1 Tablespoon Baking powder

¼ cup Olive oil

1 teaspoon Baking soda

1 teaspoon Vanilla

1 teaspoon Cinnamon

2 Eggs, beaten

1 teaspoon Ginger

½ teaspoon Sea Salt

Preheat oven to 375°. Combine flour and the next 7 ingredients in a medium bowl. Make a well in the center of the mixture. Combine pumpkin, and the next 5 ingredients. Add to the flour mixture; stir until just moist. Spoon into muffin cups, sprayed lightly with cooking spray.

Bake at 375 for 20-25 minutes or until muffins spring back when touched. Remove from oven and cool on a rack.

Stuffed Vegetables

Stuff celery with chicken, turkey, tuna, or egg salad, or peanut butter.

Stuff lettuce with any meat or egg filling and roll up.

Stuff baked potato with grated cheese, chopped broccoli, peas, chopped red bell pepper, spinach, or sour cream or Greek yogurt. (Bake potatoes, scoop out and mash insides and combine with fillings. Replace on skins and place in the oven to melt cheese.) For added protein, serve with hummus and celery, or nuts.

Soups/Chili

Use homemade or commercial, but read labels for additives, colors, sugars, flavorings, and preservatives. Enhance store bought soups by adding your own vegetables in small chunks. Add carrots, corn, or zucchini to a favorite chili recipe.

Raw Tapioca Pudding
From Anni Fiske

½ cup raw cashews
1 ½ cups water
½ tablespoon vanilla
1 tablespoon Agave (or raw honey)
1/8 teaspoon Almond extract
1 pinch of salt
1/8 cup Chia seeds

Blend water and cashews well in a blender. Add vanilla, Agave, Almond extract, and salt. Blend well. Pour into a large Mason jar and add in the Chia seeds. Cover with a lid and shake well. Let stay overnight in the refrigerator.

Vegetable Soup

2 leeks, washed well and chopped
3 garlic cloves, chopped
1 tablespoon olive oil
1 cup sliced carrots
1 cup cubed peeled acorn squash
2 sweet potatoes, cubed
1 cup chopped spinach, fresh or frozen
Wine Vinegar or Tamari soy sauce
Salt and pepper to taste

Sauté leeks and garlic in oil in a large pot until golden. Place all vegetables in boiling water, cover and cook over low heat until tender, about 30 minutes. Strain out vegetables, reserving cooking water, and puree in blender or processor. Add vegetables to cooking water; stir well, season with sauce, salt and pepper, and heat through. (You can add tomato juice or pureed tomatoes, but omit spinach.)

Vegetables, Stir-fried

2 tablespoons coconut oil
1 onion, chopped
1 leek, sliced thin
2 garlic cloves, minced
½ cup sesame seeds
2 stalks broccoli
2 carrots, chopped fine
1 sweet potato, chopped fine
2 asparagus stalks, chopped fine
1 cup shredded kale, or collards
1 red pepper, chopped fine
1 cup chopped spinach
1 cup dried shiitake mushrooms

Save time by cutting the vegetables in advance. In a wok or deep frying pan heat oil and add onion, leek, garlic, and sesame seeds. Stir with a wooden spoon continuously to brown, but not burning the garlic. Add broccoli, carrots, sweet potato, and asparagus. Stir continually for about 5 minutes. Add remaining vegetables and continue stirring until slightly tender. Add tamari or other seasonings and a bit of water if vegetables become dry. Cover and lower heat. Cook until vegetables are done; but not over cooked. Serve with brown rice or noodles. For protein, add beef, chicken or turkey.

Wheat berry Soup
From Cooking with the Bible

1 cup wheat berries
Cold water for soaking (or 4 cups boiling water as an alternative)
5 cups plain tomato sauce
1½ cups navy beans
6 new potatoes, diced
1 large onion, sliced
4 cloves garlic, minced
5 teaspoon ground cumin
1 tablespoon turmeric
½ teaspoon ground black pepper
2 green peppers, chopped

Soak the wheat berries overnight in cold water. If this is not possible, put 1 cup of wheat berries in a small pot with boiling water and simmer till all water evaporates. Berries will then be open and full.

Add berries to remaining ingredients in a large pot and cook for 1 hour on a low flame. Serve piping hot.

Yield: 8 servings

Food Labels and What do They Mean?

Organic- Strictly regulated by the government. Soil had to have no pesticides, synthetic fertilizers, or chemicals for two years. The soil is replenished rather than depleted and water systems are preserved rather than polluted. However, according to Fitzgerald, there can be traces of pesticides on organic produce for several reasons. (1) Past pesticide use leaves soil contaminated through successive growing seasons. (2) Wind carries pesticide sprays from nearby nonorganic farms. (3) Some tested samples have been mislabeled as organic, due to innocent mistakes or fraud. Deception in the organic industry is disconcerting. Many synthetic substances could be used in the production of organic foods including leavening agents, ripening agents, thickeners and others, reports Fitzgerald.[12]

Natural- That which comes from nature. Not strictly regulated. Loosely defined and is not always what it seems and doesn't mean it is healthy. High-fructose corn syrup is touted at natural because it comes from corn. But you are not eating corn; you are eating chemically processed dextrose and worse possibly, Genetically Engineered corn. And that is surely not natural.

Fresh- Should mean directly from the farm or orchard, not previously frozen or canned.

Hormone free- Poultry is free of hormones, but other meat can be contaminated. Look for "antibiotic-free" because this is used as a growth promoter and is toxic.

Free-range- Means not confined to small space. The animals are allowed to roam in an open space at will.

Grass Fed- This is a voluntary label and is regulated by the USDA for beef and lamb. It means the animal has access to pasture and was not fed grain. Look for "USDA Process Verified" and "U.S. Grass Fed on the package.

Whole grain- 100% Whole grain has twice as much fiber as "made with whole grain." Whole wheat is not the same. It is still processed and stripped of its nutrients. This is a label that is extremely deceptive. Be cautious. Cheerios is touted as 100% whole grain but it has been refined so much that has become processed. It is no longer whole grain.

Trans-fat free- A product can be called trans-fat free as long as each serving has half a gram or less. If you eat more than a single serving, you get more than half a gram. Also, any oil heated for cooking or frying turns to a trans-fat. If a product says, hydrogenated or partially hydrogenated it has trans fats.

Sources:
Russell, Natalie. *USA Weekend.* 2008
Melina, Vesanto, R.D. Becoming Vegetarian. 1995

Biblical Essential Oils
Referenced from David Stewart, PhD, *Healing Oils of the Bible*
(Used with permission.)

The references below are only a limited list of references to oils and herbs used in Biblical times.

1. **Myrrh** (Commiphora myrrha) - Increases feelings of well-being, prevents infections, insect repellant, skin conditions. Used as a perfume. Support for the endocrine and immune system. **Esther 2:12, Psalm 45:7, 8**

2. **Frankincense** (Boswellia carteri)-biblical anointing oil. Stimulates the immune system, an aid for people with cancer, depression, allergies, headache, herpes, bronchitis, and brain damage. **Leviticus 2:1, Matthew 2:11**

3. **Cedarwood** (Cedrus lebani) - was used for ritual cleansing after touching something unclean. Today used for hair loss treatment, insect repellant, TB, bronchitis, gonorrhea, acne, psoriasis. It is high in sesquiterpenes, which enhance cellular oxygen. **Leviticus 14:4, 6, 49, 51, 52**

4. **Cinnamon** (Cinnamomum verum)-Effective antibacterial and antiviral agents. It supports the immune system against cold and flu by inhaling the dust or rub on the soles of your feet. It was used to perfume beds and as an anointing oil. **Exodus 30:23**

5. **Cassia**, a cousin of Cinnamon, is a potent immune enhancer. **Psalm 45:8**

6. **Calamus** (Acorus calamus)-Rich in phenylpropanoids. Was used for anointing and phenylpropanoids. Was used for anointing and as an aromatic stimulant as well as a digestive tonic. Today it is used to relax muscle, relieve inflammation, and support the respiratory system and clear kidney congestion after intoxication. Taken orally, inhaled, or applied topically. **Song of Solomon 4:14**

7. **Galbanum** (Ferula gummosa)-Was used for anointing and as a medicine. Today it is used to treat acne, asthma, cough, indigestion, muscles aches and pains, wrinkles, wounds and to balance emotions. **Exodus 30:34**

8. **Onycha** (Styrax benzoin)-The most viscous oil, was used for anointing, as an ingredient in perfume, and as medicine. Today it is used to stimulate kidney output, treat colic, gas, and constipation. It appears to help control blood sugar. It is inhaled for sinusitis, bronchitis, cold, coughs, and sore throats. Used topically to dress wounds and irritations. **Exodus 30:34**

9. **Spikenard** (Nardos)-Modern research has found it to be beneficial in treating allergies, migraines, and nausea. It supports cardiovascular function and calms the emotions. **Mark 14:3**

10. **Hyssop** (Hyssopus officinalis)-Principle cleanser in Biblical times. Modern research has shown it beneficial for relief of anxiety, arthritis, asthma, urinary tract infections, fungal and parasitic infections, cold, flu, and wound healing. It metabolizes fat, increases perspiration, and aids detoxification. **Numbers 19:6, 8**

11. **Sandalwood** (Santalum album)-Was used to enhance meditation and as an aphrodisiac. It contains sesquiterpenes that deprogram misinformation and carry cellular O2. It is used today to enhance sleep, support female endocrine and reproductive systems, relieve urinary tract infections, insect resistance, and for skin care. (Although I couldn't find specific use of Sandalwood oil, the plant existed in ancient times. It was used for trade as early as 700 BC.)

12. **Myrtle** (Myrtus communis)-Was used for purification ceremonies in Biblical times. Myrtle is used today to balance hormones, soothe the respiratory system, battle colds and flu, and treat asthma, bronchitis, coughs, and skin conditions. **Nehemiah 8:15**

13. **Cypress** (Cupressus sempervirens)-Ancient healers used the oil

to treat arthritis, laryngitis, swollen scar tissue, and cramps. Today it is used to support the cardiovascular and circulatory system and promote emotional well-being, especially in times of stress. It also promotes the production of red blood cells and boosts natural defenses. It is generally massaged along the spine, armpits, feet, heart, and chest. **1 Kings 6:34**

14. **Rose of Sharon** (Cistus ladanifer)-Used historically as a mood elevator. Today it is used as an antiseptic, immune enhancer, and nerve calmative. **Solomon 2:1**

Common Herbs of the Bible
Referenced from *Herbs of the Bible* by James Duke, Ph.D., 2007

Listed below are some of the most researched and commonly used herbs. Some of the scriptural references are noted. The herbs are listed as a reference only and are not intended to diagnose or treat any diseases or to be used in place of standard medical care. Please speak to your doctor before using any herbs if you are on medication or currently experiencing a health disorder.

Aloe Vera

• Several forms were used in the Bible. Aloes come from a tree in China and India. The seeds contain the oil. The aloes in biblical references were not the typical American aloe. Aloe is known to soothe burns and other skin irritations. It is also effective for healing the stomach and lower intestines. Can be applied internally or externally. **John 19:39-40**

Anise

• This spice resembled caraway and was used as a seasoning. **Matthew 23:23**

Black Cumin (Nigella sativa)

- Commonly used in breads and cakes or to purge the body of worms and parasites. It is helpful as an antihistamine effect on asthma, bronchitis and coughs. **Isaiah 28:25**

Black Mustard (Brassica nigra)

- Grew along the Sea of Galilee. It contains both fixed and essential oil. It has been used as a plaster for arthritis and rheumatism. Useful for congestion in head afflictions, neuralgia, or muscle spasm. **Luke 13:19**

Cinnamon (Cinnamomum verum)

- Part of the holy anointing oil used to anoint priests and vessels in the tabernacle of Moses in Exodus 30:22-25. It calms the stomach and may prevent ulcers. It can alleviate indigestion, stomach cramps, intestinal spasms, nausea and flatulence, improve appetite and help with diarrhea. The extracts are active against Candida albicans, the fungus responsible for yeast infections.[17] Cinnamon contains benzaldehyde, an anti-tumor agent, also having antiseptic properties that kill the bacteria that cause tooth decay. It has been known to be useful as a food preservative to inhibit the growth of common food-borne bacteria such as Salmonella and E.coli.[17] Helps stabilize blood sugar in Type II diabetes. One-eighth teaspoon triples insulin efficiency. **Proverbs 7:17-18**

Coriander (Corindrum sativum)

- Also known as: Cilantro and Chinese parsley. Used for acid indigestion, gas, neuralgia, rheumatism, and toothaches. It contains 20 natural antibacterial chemicals that help control body odor. **Numbers 11:7**

Cucumber

- Grown along the Nile, it was a cooling fruit enjoyed in Egypt during the summer heat. **Isaiah 1:8**

Dandelion (Taraxicum offininale)

- One of the bitter herbs eaten at Passover. Traditionally used as a remedy for cancer, diabetes, hepatitis, osteoporosis, and rheumatism. Has a safe diuretic effect and is high in Vitamin C and beta-carotene. It is a powerful purgative for the kidney and liver. **Numbers 9:11**

Dill (Athenum graveolens)

- It was valuable in ancient Israel and the Israelites were required to tithe with it from their supplies. Research supports the 3,000 year old use as a digestive aid and for excessive intestinal gas. Dill seed oil inhibits the growth of several digestive tract bacteria.

Fenugreek (Trigonella fenum-graecum)

- Referred to as Leeks in the Bible. Long considered a "cure all." Research has identified five compounds in the seeds that help diabetics lower blood sugar. **Numbers 11:5**

Frankincense (Boswellia sacra)

- One of the gifts of the Magi to the baby Jesus. One of the four exclusive components used to make holy incense for the tabernacle of Moses. It is still used by the Roman Catholic Church. Common offerings. **Matthew 2:11; Nehemiah 13:5; Exodus 30:34; Leviticus 24:7; Song of Solomon 3:6; Matthew 2:11**

Garlic (Allium sativum)

- Effective infection fighter, mosquito and tick repellant. It is an antibacterial and antiviral.[17] It has pain killing properties as well as being an immune stimulant. Also useful for high blood pressure, asthma, fungus, parasites, yeast, and diabetes. **Numbers 11:5**

Henna (Lawsonia inermis)

- Historically used as cosmetics and hair dye. It contains the chemical lawsone, an active antibiotic and fungicide often used for fungal infections of the nails.**Solomon 4:13**

Hyssop (Hyssop officinalis or Origganum syriacum)

- Also known as: Marjoram/Capers. It is a spice, a tonic, and a digestive aid. It was used for spreading blood on the doorposts for Passover. Capers are the berries of the plant. It stops bleeding, masks odors, a digestive aid, cold remedy and anti-inflammatory. **Exodus 12:22; Numbers 19:6, 18; 1 Kings 4:33; Psalm 51:7**

Juniper (Juniperus oxycedrus)

- Conifer under growth found in Israel. It was probably the "algum" timber King Solomon requested of Hirum, king of Tyre. It has been used for skin parasites in animals, psoriasis, eczema, as well as other skin and scalp conditions. It appears to inhibit viruses linked with cold and flu. **2 Chronicles 2:8**

Leek

- Leeks seem to be used synonymously with onion in biblical references. They are good for throat disorders and acute nasal discharges due to their ability to loosen phlegm. Leeks are also good blood purifiers and general immune stimulating as well as helpful to the respiratory and cardiovascular systems.[20]

Milk Thistle (Silymarin marianum)

- Has been used as a liver remedy since biblical times. It contains silymarin, a natural, powerful compound that prevents repairs and even regenerates the liver. It also has been shown to lower blood sugar and insulin levels in diabetics and help prevent gallstones. The seeds contain eight anti-inflammatory compounds that aid in healing skin conditions and infections. **Job 31:40**

Mint or Horsemint (Mentha longifolia)

- Sweet scented plants mentioned in the Bible are found in **Matthew 23:23** and **Luke 11:42**. Some species have been effective with Alzheimer's disease, aid digestion, and is an anti-allergenic. The oil is used in aromatherapy to stimulate brain activity.

Myrrh (Cistus inasus or Commiphora erythreae)

- One hundred thirty-three varieties found in the Middle East. Used for purification. **Esther 2:12; Psalm 45:8** It has been used as an anti-bacterial mouthwash, and bronchial infections. Myrrh contains furanosequeterpenoid, a chemical compound that kills cells resistant to chemotherapy and in some cancers.

Nettle (Urtica dioica)

- Stinging Nettle. Has been used to eliminate arthritis. It is a rich source of Vitamins A, C, and E as well as many anti-oxidants. **Job 30:7**

Onion

- Although not an herb, it has healing properties. It is known to relieve congestion, reduce inflammation, lower blood pressure, inhibit allergic, inflammatory responses. Onions contain sulfides similar to garlic that can lower blood lipids. They are a rich source of flavonoids that provide protection against cardiovascular disease due to the anti-clotting agents. **Numbers 11:5**

Pomegranate

- Not an herb, rather a fruit with many healing properties. **Deuteronomy 8:8; Joel 1:12**

Saffron (Crocus sativus)

- It was the world's most expensive herb in biblical times. One ounce requires 4,300 flowers. Saffron has been used for gastric and intestinal problems and is considered an anti-spasmodic, an expectorant, a sedative and a stimulant. **Solomon 4:14**

Sage (Lampstand)

- Used as a perfume and for medicinal purposes. **Exodus 37:17, 18**

Spikenard (Nardostachys grandiflora or jatamansi)

- Remember the woman that anointed Jesus with the spikenard from her alabaster jar, which cost a year's wages? It is used as a stimulant, for epilepsy, hysteria, heart palpitations, and chorea. Spikenard oil may help auricular flutter, and depress the Central Nervous System as well as relax skeletal muscles. **Mark 14:3**

Biblical Reference Chart to Common Illnesses of Ancient Times (Used for reference only)

Illness	Herb/Essential Oil Remedy	Biblical Reference
Fever	Cucumber	De. 28:22, Ma. 8:14, Nu. 11:4-6
Dysentery	Cinnamon (Antibacterial), aloe, coriander	2 Chron, 21:12-19, Ex. 30:23, Jo. 19:39
Leprosy	Cedarwood	Lev. 13:2, 14:4, 6, 2 Ki. 5:1
Intestinal worms	Cumin, dill, aloe, fennel	Acts 12:23, Is. 28:25-27, Ma. 23:23, Jo. 19:39-40
Plague	Frankincense, cinnamon, clove, garlic	Nu. 11:33, 2 Sam. 24:15, Lev. 2:1
Paralysis		Ma. 2:24
Epilepsy, muscle spasms	Eucalyptus, frankincense, black mustard, spikenard	Ma. 8:6, Ma. 9:2
Digestive upset	Ginger	
Insanity		Ma. 4:24
Opthalmia	Fennel (diluted), cumin, raw honey	
Skin disorders	Cedarwood, galbanum, sandalwood, myrtle, aloe, juniper, pomegranate	Job 2:7-10, 2 Ki. 20:7, De. 28:27, Lu. 16:20, Lev. 14:4, 6, 49, 51-52, Ex. 30:34, Ne. 8:15, Jo. 19:39-40, 2 Chron. 2:8-9, Sol. 8:2, Ps. 105:31
Faint		Dan. 8:27
Atrophy		Job 19:20
Blind	Mud pack	Job 29:15, Jo. 9:6

Deaf		Ps. 38:13, Mk. 7:32
Dropsy		Lu. 14:2
Hemorrhage		Ma. 9:20
Lame	Dandelion	Nu. 9:11, 2 Chron. 16:12
Infections	Myrrh, frankincense, hyssop	Esth. 2:12, Ps. 45:7 8, Lev. 2:1, Nu. 19:6, 8
	Anointing	Mk. 6:13, Ja. 5:14
	Laid in streets for advice	Mk. 6:56, Acts 5:15
	Divinely supported	Ps. 41:3
	Divinely cured	2Ki. 20:5
Liver/Blood purifier	Chicory, leeks, milk thistle	Nu. 9:11, Job 31:40
Medicinal herb	Dandelion	Ex. 12:8
	Endive	Gen. 2:5
	Sorrel	Ex. 9:25
Snakebites	Fennel	
Digestive tonic	Calamus, onycha, galbanum, aloe, cinnamon, coriander, mint, saffron	Sol. 4:14, Ex. 30:34, Jo. 19:39-40, Ps. 45:8, Nu. 11:7, Ex. 16:31, Ma. 23:23
Immune support	Frankincense, cedarwood, cinnamon, cassia, onycha, garlic	Lev. 2:1, Lev. 14:4, 6, Ex. 30:23, Ps. 45:8, Ex. 30:34, Prov. 7:17-18, Nu. 11:5
Inflammation	Cypress, black mustard, milk thistle, nettle, onion, leeks	1 Ki. 6:34, Lu. 13:19, Job 31:40, Job 30:7, Nu. 11:5
Wounds, burns	Galbanum, myrrh, honey, lavender, ginger, cedar	Ex. 30:34, Esth. 2:12, Ps. 45:7-8
Emotions	Spikenard, hyssop, rose of sharon	Mk. 14:3, Nu. 19:6, 8, Sol. 2:1
Brain Stimulant	Mint	Lu. 11:42, Ma. 23:23

RESOURCES

www.apexenergetics.com   (Please call for a health care practitioner in your local area associated with the company to order products.)

www.azurestandard.com   (CSA food Co-op. Contact the company to find a local drop off in your area.)

www.biblesearch.com

www.biokleen.com (for pure laundry soap and dish detergent)

www.bobsredmill.com (100% whole grain flours and gluten free flours)

www.celiacdiseasefoundation.org

www.cookingwiththebible.com

www.glutensolutions.com

www.greenpasture.org   (organic coconut oil)

www.hallelujahacres.com

www.heavenlyorganics.com

www.individualizedwellness.net

www.livingfuel.com   (whole food protein shakes and bars)

www.prlabs.com(Please call Premier Research Labs for a health care practitioner in your local area associated with the company to order products.)

www.slowfoodusa.org

www.westonapricefoundation.org(Contact the company for a local chapter dairy Co-op)

BIBLIOGRAPHY

1. Adams, Mike. *Pasteurized milk 150 times more contaminated with blood, pus and feces than fresh milk - videos the CDC won't show you.* Natural News: February 22, 2012

2. Batmanghelidj, F. M.D. *You're Not Sick, You're Thirsty!* New York, New York. Warner Books, Inc., 2003

3. Burk, Dean, M.D. *Cancer Deaths Linked to Water Fluoridation.* February 4, 2012. www.orthomolecular.org/library/jom. 2001

4. Carlisle, Paul. *With All My Heart God's Design for Emotional Wellness,* 2000.

5. Cherniske, Stephen. *Caffeine Blues: Wake UP to the Hidden Dangers of America's #1 Drug.* New York: Warner, 1998.

6. Colbert, Don, M.D. *Seven Pillars of Health.* Lake Mary, Florida: Siloam Pub., 2006

7. Colbert, Don, M.D. *Toxic Relief.* Lake Mary, Florida: Siloam Pub., 1984

8. Colquhoun, James and Ten Bosch, Laurentine. *FoodMatters, You are What You Eat,* Permacology Productions, 2008

9. Cordain, Loren, PhD. *The Origin and Evolution of the Western Diet.* January 2012

10. Davies, Lorene-Cron. *Sol Salt for Health,* 2007

11. *Eight Laws of Health,* Bottom Line Health, January 2009:35

12. Fitzgerald, Randall. *The Hundred Year Lie.* New York, New York: Dutton, 2006.

13. Freston, Kathy. *Quantum Wellness*. New York, New York: Weinstein Books, 2007

14. Frost, Mary, M.A. *Going Back To the Basics of Human Health.*

15. Geary, Mike. *The Canola Oil Marketing Deception -Have you been lied to about the health benefits of canola oil?* 2012

16. Gianni, Kevin. *Keeping Your Bones Healthy Isn't All About Calcium*, Exclusive Renegade Health Article, Dec. 6, 2011

17. *Harmful Ingredients Found in Children's Vitamins.* Health Keepers Magazine, December 2011:21, 29

18. Heneman, Karrie, PhD. *Some Facts about Energy Drinks, Nutrition and Health Info-sheet*, U.C. Davis Cooperative Extension, 2007

19. Hoffer, Abram, M.D. *Putting It All Together: The New Orthomolecular Nutrition.* Keats Publishing, 1978

20. Jensen, Bernard, M.D. *Foods That Heal.* Garden City, NY: Avery Pub., 1993

21. Kneebone, William, DC, CNC, DiHom. *Biblically Based Health Strategies for Christians*

22. Lawrence, Cameron. *Fasting and Feasting: Finding the necessary Balance.* In Touch, November 2011

23. Leaf, Caroline, PhD. *The Mind is What the Brain Does...and Coffee Helps.* www.drleaf.com/index.php: January 24, 2012.

24. Ludwig, Garth D. *Order Restored*, 1999.

25. Malinauskas, Brenda. *A Survey of Energy Drink Consumption Patterns among College Students.* Nutrition Journal, 2007, 6:35

26. Marshall, Robert, PhD. Premier Research Labs, 2007

27. Mercola, Joseph, M.D. *Refuse to Eat These Foods—They Could Destroy Your Reproductive Organs.* January 10, 2012

28. Mercola, Joseph, M.D. Reuters, April 29,1004

29. Nagel, Ramie. *Cure Tooth Decay.* Golden Child Publishing, 2011

30. Pink, Arthur. *The Attributes of God,* Wilder Publications, 2008

31. Pink, Arthur. *Sayings of Christ on the Cross.*

32. Polk, Brenda. *With All My Strength God's Design for Physical Wellness,* 2002

33. Pollan, Michael. *In Defense of Food: an Eater's Manifesto.* New York: Penguin, 2008

34. Pollan, Michael. *Food Rules.* New York: Penguin Press, 2011

35. Price, Weston A., *Nutrition and Physical Degeneration.* Medical Book Department of Harper and Brothers, 1939

36. Pottenger, Francis. *Pottenger's Cats.* La Mesa, CA: Price-Pottenger Nutrition Foundation, 1983

37. Rapp, Doris J. *Our Toxic World.* Environmental Medical Research Foundation, 2004

38. Rodier, Hugo, M.D. *Sweet Death, The Epidemic That's Killing America,* 2007

39. Rubin, Jordan. *The Maker's Diet.* Lake Mary, FL: Siloam, 2004

40. Ruvolo, Carol J. *A Believer's Guide to Spiritual Fitness.* P & R Publishing, 2000

41. Ryrie, Charles Caldwell. ThD., Ph.D. *The Ryrie Study Bible,* 1985.

42. Safer, Morley. *The Flavorists.* CBS 60 Minutes, Nov. 27, 2011

43. Schlosser, Eric. *Fast Food Nation.* Boston, New York: Houghton Mifflin Company, 2001

44. Schwartzbein, Diane, M.D. *The Schwartzbein Principle.* Health Communications, Inc., 2002

45. Stanley, Charles. *In Touch.* October 2011

46. Stanley, Charles. *In Touch.* March 2012

47. Stanley, Charles. *Wisdom's Way.* 2001

48. Staessen, Jan A. MD, PhD. *Author Insights: Questioning the Benefits of Salt Restriction,* news@JAMA, May 3, 2011

49. Stewart, David. *Healing Oils of the Bible.* Marble Hill, MO: Care Publications, 2003

50. Stiteler, Stephen. *Coffee-It's Time to Avoid It!* 2002

51. *Switch to Low Fat,* USA Weekend, October 2011

52. Wartman, Kristin, CNE. *Not Your Grandma's Milk,* www. kristinwartman.wordpress.com, 2011

53. White, Ellen Gould Harmon. *Selected Messages.* Hagerstown, MD: Review and Herald, 2006

54. Williams, Debbie Taylor. *If God is in Control, Why Do I Have a Headache?* 2004

55. Winnail, Douglas S. *Defeating Disease: How the Bible Can Help.* Tomorrow's World: 2006

56. www.bibleclassics.com

57. www.ehow.com/erythritol

58. www.en.wikipedia.org

59. www.jvi.asm.org/cgi/content/full/76/22/11321

60. www.kew.org/plant-cultures/plants/sandalwood

61. www.lewismountain.ca/sauerkraut_history.html

62. www.medicine.net

63. www.myadrenalfatigue.com/energydrinks

64. www.ncbi.nim.nih.gov/pubmed/22118754#. *Combination of erythritol and fructose increases gastrointestinal symptoms in healthy adults.* Nutrition Research, November 2011: 31(11): 836-41

65. www.olympic.org/ancient-olympic-games

66. www.robbwolf.com

67. www.uhn.edu/msa/pork.htm

68. www.wikipedia/salt

69. www.wikipedia/iodine